Bone
Histomorphometry

Bone Histomorphometry

Erik Fink Eriksen *M.D., Dr. Med. Sci.*
Assistant Professor of Medicine
University Department of Endocrinology
Aarhus Amtssygehus
Aarhus, Denmark

Douglas W. Axelrod *M.D., Ph. D.*
Medical Director
Bone and Mineral Research
Proctor & Gamble Pharmaceuticals
Norwich, New York

Flemming Melsen *M.D., Ph. D.*
Professor of Medicine
University Department of Pathology
Aarhus Amtssygehus
Aarhus, Denmark

Raven Press New York

Raven Press, Ltd., 1185 Avenue of the Americas, New York, New York 10036

Printed and bound in Hong Kong

Library of Congress Cataloging-in-Publication Data

Eriksen, Erik Fink.
    Bone Histomorphometry/Erik Fink Eriksen, Douglas W. Axelrod, Flemming Melsen.
        p. cm.
    Includes bibliographical references and index
    ISBN 0-7817-0122-8
    1. Bone–Histology. 2. Bone–Histopathology. 3. Bone remodeling. I. Axelrod, Douglas W. II. Melsen, Flemming. III. Title.
    [DNLM: 1. Bone Remodeling–physiology. 2. Bone and Bones–anatomy & histology. 3. Bone Diseases, Metabolic–physiopathology. WE 200 E69 1994]
    QM569. E69 1994
    611'.0184–dc20
    DNLM/DLC
    for Library of Congress   93-24476
                                               CIP

9 8 7 6 5 4 3 2 1

CONTENTS

ASBMR Sponsorship Statement... vii

Preface ix

Acknowledgments xi

1   **Skeletal Growth, Modeling, and Remodeling** 1

2   **Bone Macroanatomy and Microanatomy** 3
    Cortical bone 3
    Cancellous bone 6
    Lamellar and woven bone 7
    Summary 12

3   **The Cellular Basis of Bone Remodeling** 13
    The remodeling sequence in cortical bone 13
    The remodeling sequence in cancellous bone 14
    Activation frequency 15
    The quantum concept of bone remodeling 15
    Summary 20

4   **Bone Remodeling and Changes in Bone Mass** 21
    Reversible changes in bone mass 21
    Irreversible changes in bone mass 22
    Summary 28

5   **Bone Remodeling and Bone Mass Measurements** 29
    Summary 31

6   **Bone Histology and Histomorphometry** 33
    The basis for histomorphometric evaluation 33
    Indications for bone biopsy 35

Bone biopsy procedures and sample
  preparation techniques 35
Summary 38

7 Histomorphometric Indices 39
Primary and secondary histomorphometric indices 39
Cell number 41
Surface estimates 41
Erosion and formation periods 43
Activation frequency 43
Tissue-level volume-referent indices 43
Reconstruction of the remodeling sequence 44
Key indices of bone remodeling and bone balance 44
Regional acceleratory phenomenon 47
Summary 48

8 Bone Structure and Bone Strength 49

9 Bone Remodeling in Metabolic Bone Disease 51
Osteoporosis 51
Osteomalacia 54
Thyroid disorders 55
Primary and secondary hyperparathyroidism 55
Corticosteroid-induced osteopenia 59

References 61

Index 69

ASBMR Sponsorship Statement

We are pleased to introduce this edition of *Bone Histomorphometry*. As the bone and mineral sciences have grown rapidly in recent years, so too have new techniques that further our understanding of bone metabolism and its role in health and disease. Important among these are the techniques of bone histomorphometry.

From the pioneering work of Frost through the efforts of many contemporary researchers, bone histomorphometry has evolved into a tool that provides valuable insights into the function and dysfunction of bone. This monograph integrates fundamental concepts of the cellular basis of the bone remodeling with the methods of histomorphometric analysis, providing a foundation for understanding bone dynamics and improving diagnostic and therapeutic interventions.

The American Society of Bone and Mineral Research is pleased to endorse this monograph, which will serve as an introductory manual for students new to the field as well as a reference guide for those already within the field.

Murray J. Favus, M.D.
Education Comittee, ASBMR

Bone science is undergoing a surge of activity, motivated by (1) new understandings of bone biology, (2) new tools with which to investigate bone physiology, and (3) new therapeutic agents to control the pathophysiologic processes. It is now clear that an understanding of basic bone biology is necessary to best understand and intervene in important metabolic bone diseases, such as osteoporosis and Paget's disease of bone.

Bone histomorphometry is an actively evolving tool with which to gain insight into the processes of normal and abnormal bone physiology. Beyond providing a qualitative view of bone at the microscopic level, histomorphometric techniques now enable us to understand the kinetics of bone turnover and quantify the changes in bone balance at the cellular level. Some of the newest advances also allow us to gain information about the three-dimensional structure of bone, using indices such as the marrow star volume.

It is the intent of this book to impart to the practitioner a basic understanding of bone biology, which is necessary to employ the tool of histomorphometry in the practice of medicine, and, in so doing, to facilitate informed diagnostic and therapeutic decisions.

E.F. Eriksen, M.D., Dr. Med. Sci.
D.W. Axelrod, M.D., Ph.D.
F. Melsen, M.D., Ph.D.

ACKNOWLEDGMENTS

We wish to thank our coworkers and colleagues for their support. Special thanks are extended to our colleagues at the Aarhus Bone and Mineral Research Center for their exemplary research and work in preparing and photographing the numerous biopsy sections used to illustrate this monograph. We also wish to thank Professor A.M. Parfitt, Professor R.R. Recker, and Professor R.E. Canfield for their constructive reviews of earlier versions of this monograph.

We particularly wish to thank P.J. (Cilla) Davis, Editor in the Life Sciences, whose perspicacity and drive for editorial excellence improved this document enormously and without whom this project would not likely have come to fruition.

Lastly, we acknowledge our fellow researchers in the field of bone and mineral research whose ingenious efforts to elucidate the mysteries of living bone proved to be the catalyst to our efforts. The more we know, the more we seek to discover. We would be grateful to hear of any suggestions or additions that might be considered for future editions.

Bone
Histomorphometry

Skeletal Growth, Modeling, and Remodeling

On a macroscopic level, the skeleton can change size or shape or simply renew old structures without changing shape. Each of these processes may employ different mechanisms, with different controlling influences.

Growth of the skeleton in childhood and adolescence takes place at growth plates, areas in which cartilage proliferates and gradually undergoes calcification, leading to longitudinal growth. This growth occurs mainly in the cartilage compartment of the epiphyseal and metaphyseal areas of long bones. The growing cartilage gradually becomes calcified, thus forming primary new bone. In this way, centers of proliferating cartilage can produce overall bone growth.

Bone modeling is the process is by which the overall shape of bone is changed in response to physiologic and/or mechanical influences. Bone may widen or change in axis by the removal or addition of bone. For example, an increase in the width of long bones is caused by the addition of new layers of bone at the periosteal surface while removal of bone occurs at the endosteal surface. Wolff's Law, that long bones change shape to accommodate the lines of stress, is a hypothesis based on the modeling of bone.

Bone remodeling is the life-long process by which bone is renewed through the continuous removal of bone (bone resorption) and the replacement of discrete amounts of old bone by the synthe-

1

sis of new bone matrix and its subsequent mineralization (bone formation). This activity has been extensively characterized, in particular through the understanding of the cellular and spatial components in which this activity occurs.

On a macroscopic level, remodeling may not be evident over time, as long as the removal and replacement phases are balanced. On a microscopic level, remodeling is an active process throughout the skeleton and is mediated through the coupled processes of bone resorption and bone formation. By these coupled processes, the mechanical integrity of the skeleton is preserved. Moreover, together with the kidneys and the gut, bone remodeling is an integral part of the calcium homeostasic system. Removal of old bone leads to the liberation of calcium to serve metabolic needs. The release of bone constituents into the serum is also the basis for the determination of calcium kinetics and the use of matrix degradation products as biochemical markers of bone resorption.

The cells that remodel bone act within the framework of the basic multicellular unit (BMU) (1) or bone remodeling unit (BRU) (2). Although there are slight differences in the definitions of these units, the term BRU will be used for the remainder of this discussion. Over time, this multicellular cohort effects the resorption of old bone and the formation of new bone to replace it. The BRU may take different forms in different types of bone but remains the stereotypic instrument by which bone is remodeled. The end result of a remodeling cycle in an individual BRU is the bone structural unit (BSU) (1, 2, 3).

Disturbances in bone remodeling can lead to alterations in bone architecture. The removal of structural elements in bone is followed by a loss of mechanical competence and a subsequent increase in the risk of skeletal fracture. Restoration of bone structure and mechanical competence can be achieved only if these processes are reversed by treatment regimens that create a positive bone balance and restore bone architecture. A thorough understanding of bone remodeling is therefore very important, not only in relation to clinical decision-making in metabolic bone disease but also in the interpretation of serum bone marker levels, bone mass measurements, and calcium kinetic indices. Thus, an understanding of bone remodeling and histomorphometric analysis constitutes the very basis for the design and implementation of more effective treatments for metabolic bone diseases.

Bone Macroanatomy and Microanatomy

The skeleton consists of two macroscopically different types of bone: *cortical bone*, which predominates in the long bones of the extremities (the appendicular skeleton), and *cancellous bone* (also known as trabecular bone), which predominates in the vertebrae and pelvis (the axial skeleton) (Fig. 1).

Cortical bone makes up 80% of the mass of the skeleton, with cancellous bone constituting the remaining 20%. However, because cancellous bone is metabolically more active per unit volume, skeletal metabolism is approximately equally distributed between the two types of bone (2). It is important to appreciate that cortical and cancellous bone behave differently and exhibit different responses to metabolic changes and treatment. The quantitative features of cortical and cancellous bone are described in Table 1.

CORTICAL BONE

Cortical bone is compact, dense bone, such as that seen in the shafts of long bones and in the vertebral endplates. It is remodeled through the activity of bone remodeling units (BRUs). The BRU in cortical bone is approximately 400 mm long and 200 mm wide at the base. In dogs, it moves longitudinally through the cortex at a rate of 40 mm/day (4). An individual BRU bores through the bone as a "cutting cone," leaving new bone behind (the "closing cone") (Fig. 2). When completed, this "haversian system" (or cortical osteon) consists of lamellae arranged in concentric layers along the

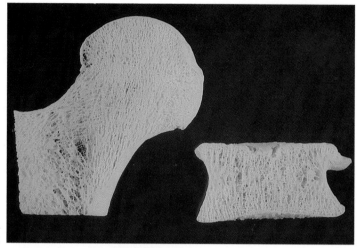

FIG. 1. Cortical and cancellous bone as seen in cross-sections of femur and vertebra in macerated preparations (**a**) and on contact radiographs (**b**). Note the preferential orientation of trabeculae.

BRU's long axis around a central (haversian) canal containing blood vessels (Fig. 2). The cortical osteon constitutes a bone structural unit (BSU), representing the end result of a remodeling cycle in cortical bone.

Provided skeletal size and turnover are normal, a total of 21 x 10⁶ BSUs will be present (Table 1); the total area (i.e., the total internal surface) available for haversian remodeling amounts to 3.5 m² (2). The porosity of cortical bone is usually less than 5%, as a result of either ongoing remodeling or the presence of the haversian canals of resting osteons. If remodeling activity increases, an increase in porosity and a decrease in cortical bone mass may be expected.

Cortical bone may itself be divided into two functional and anatomic types: periosteal and endosteal. The *periosteal* surface of cortical bone is important in appositional growth and fracture repair. It displays an imbalance between bone formation and resorption such that a net increase in bone occurs with time. In long bones, this also accounts for a net increase in diameter over time. Certain drugs, such as prostaglandin E$_2$, may elicit exaggerated periosteal bone formation. The *endosteal* surface of cortical bone, which amounts to 0.5 m² (2), has a higher level of remodeling activity, likely resulting from more mechanical strain and/or the proximity of the marrow space with its own cytokine environment. On the endosteal surfaces, resorption tends to exceed formation, leading to expansion of the marrow space in long bones. This endocortical thinning

TABLE 1. *Quantitative features of cortical and cancellous bone*

Index	Cortical bone	Cancellous bone
Fraction of skeleton (%)	80	20
Fraction of skeletal turnover (%)	50	50
Fractional tissue volume (mm³/ mm³)	0.95	0.20
Surface-to-bone volume ratio (mm²/ mm³)	2.5	20
Total bone volume (mm³)	1.4×10^6	0.35×10^6
Total internal surface (mm²)	3.5×10^6	7.0×10^6
BSU length (mm)	2.5	1.0
Wall thickness (mm)	0.04 - 0.06	0.04 - 0.06
Total number of BSUs in skeleton	21×10^6	14×10^6
Fraction of surface undergoing resorption (%)	2	4
Fraction of surface undergoing formation (%)	8	16
Fraction of quiescent surface (%)	90	80

Adapted from Parfitt (2). BSU, bone structural unit.

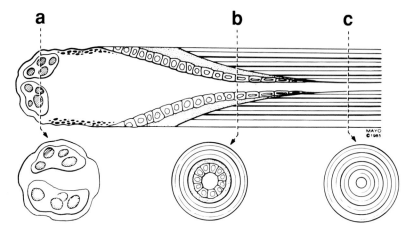

FIG. 2. The activity of the bone remodeling unit (BRU) in cortical bone as seen in longitudinal sequence and cross sections. Osteoclasts dig out a tunnel, creating a "cutting cone" (**a**). Subsequently, new bone is formed in the area of the "closing cone" (**b**), leading to the creation of a new bone structural unit (BSU) (i.e., cortical osteon or "haversian system") (**c**). From Eriksen (3). By permission of The Mayo Foundation.

may be especially pronounced during high turnover states, for example, in thyrotoxicosis and early menopause.

CANCELLOUS BONE

Cancellous bone consists of bony trabeculae, thin plates, or spicules, with thicknesses ranging from 50 mm to 400 mm. These trabeculae are interconnected in a honeycomb pattern, thereby providing maximal mechanical strength (Fig. 1). In areas subjected to mechanical stresses, the cancellous pattern develops into a structure that ensures maximal adaptation to the given stress pattern. For example, the trabecular architecture of the femoral neck mirrors the lines of stress developed during the mechanical loading produced by weight bearing (Fig. 1).

In cancellous bone, the BRU can be viewed as a cortical BRU cut longitudinally in the middle (Fig. 3). In three-dimensional terms, it constitutes a disk-like, semilunar structure, approximately 300 mm in width and several times as long (5). Cancellous BRUs resorb and form bone on the trabecular surface and, as in cortical bone, leave behind units of new lamellar bone. After the resorptive and formative phases, the resulting new bone may be observed as a wall

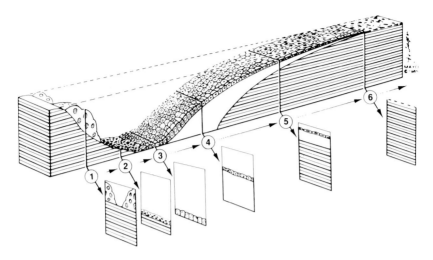

FIG. 3. The activity of the bone remodeling unit (BRU) in cancellous bone as seen in longitudinal sequence and cross sections. The BRU in cancellous bone can be viewed as a cortical BRU cut in half. Five different phases can be distinguished over time: osteoclastic resorption (**1**), mononuclear resorption (**2**), preosteoblastic migration and differentiation into osteoblasts (**3**), osteoblastic matrix (osteoid) formation (**4**), and mineralization (**5**). The end product of remodeling in cancellous bone is the completed cancellous bone structural unit (BSU) (i.e., trabecular osteon, wall or "packet" of bone) covered by lining cells (**6**). From Eriksen (3). By permission of The Mayo Foundation.

or "packet" of bone, i.e., the trabecular osteon, which is the BSU representing the end result of a remodeling cycle in cancellous bone.

The total number of these trabecular osteons has been estimated to be 14×10^6, and the total area of the trabecular surface is about 7 m^2 (Table 1) (2). Thus, in contrast with cortical bone, cancellous bone has a relatively large surface involved in remodeling activity. This explains the higher metabolic activity of cancellous bone.

LAMELLAR AND WOVEN BONE

When studying cortical or cancellous bone in polarized light, a clear lamellar pattern is visible (Fig.4). This pattern is caused by birefringence due to the arrangement of collagen fibrils in alternating orientations. The mechanism underlying this alternating orientation of fibrils is unknown, but it is clear that such a "plywood-like" orientation increases the strength of bone.

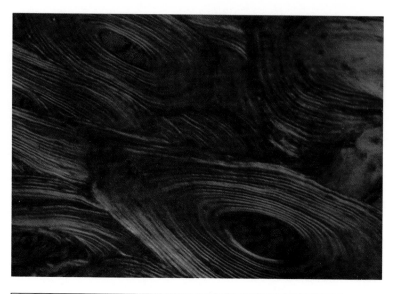

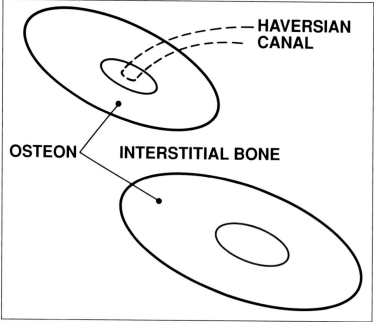

FIG. 4. Lamellar pattern of cortical (**a**) and cancellous (**b**) bone, as seen in biopsy sections studied in polarized light. Unstained, x 200.

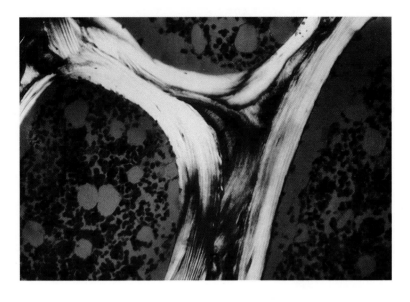

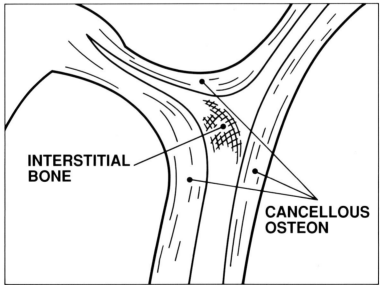

FIG. 4. Continued.

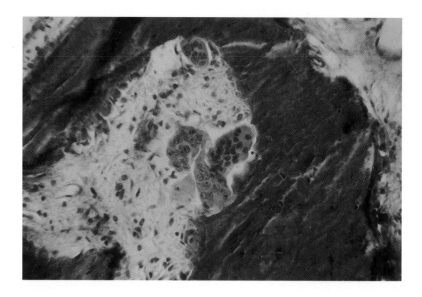

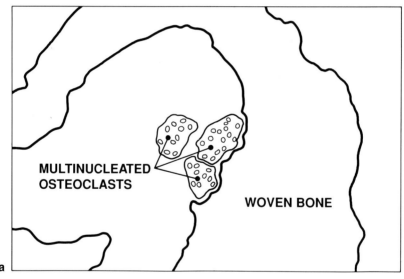

FIG. 5. Bone biopsy sections from a patient with Paget's disease of bone (**a**) and a patient receiving fluoride therapy (**b**). In **a**, note the large extremely multinucleated osteoclasts, marrow fibrosis, woven bone formation, and increased vascularization. High doses of fluoride can produce woven bone (**b**), shown here surrounding older lamellar bone. **a**, Masson-Trichrome, x 500; **b**, Masson-Trichrome, x 200.

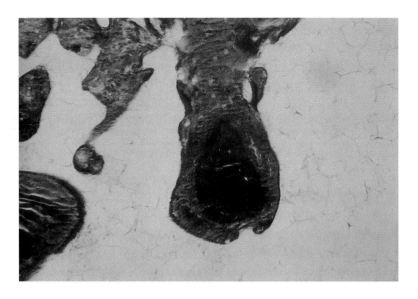

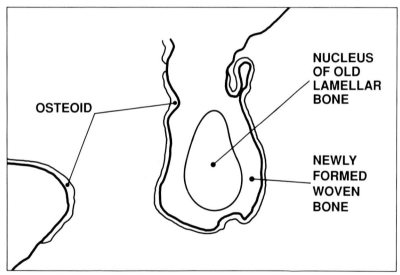

FIG. 5. Continued.

In woven bone, the lamellar pattern is absent. The collagen fibrils are laid down in a disorganized manner, and the mechanical properties of the bone therefore suffer. Woven bone is formed during the formation of primary bone or in states of high bone turnover, such as occur in Paget's disease of bone (Fig. 5a). The formation of woven bone may also occur during certain stages of fluoride treatment, in which an initial high rate of bone formation may compromise the ability of the remodeling unit to ensure proper lamellar alignment (Fig. 5b).

SUMMARY

Bone remodeling ensures the life-long renewal of the skeleton and is important for the exchange of calcium between bone and blood.

The groups of cells that remodel bone are called *bone remodeling units* (BRUs).

Cortical bone makes up 80% of the skeleton and *cancellous* (or trabecular) bone, 20%; however, because of its higher metabolic activity, cancellous bone accounts for 50% of the metabolic activity of bone.

The bone remodeling unit (BRU) of *cortical bone* creates an advancing tunnel with a "cutting cone" of resorption and a "*closing cone*" of formation of new bone (Fig. 2).

The bone remodeling unit (BRU) of *cancellous bone* resorbs and forms bone in a disk-like, semilunar structure on the surface of trabeculae (Fig. 3).

The bone structural unit (BSU) represents the end result of a remodeling cycle; in cortical bone, it constitutes a haversian system (or *cortical osteon*), and in cancellous bone, it is a wall or "packet" of bone (or *trabecular osteon*).

In *normal cortical or cancellous bone*, collagen fibrils are arranged with alternating orientation to give a clear *lamellar pattern* when viewed under polarized light; this "plywood-like" orientation increases the strength of the bone.

In *woven bone* (which may be formed as primary bone or in states of high bone turnover), collagen fibrils are arranged in a *disorganized orientation* that compromises the strength of the bone.

The Cellular Basis of Bone Remodeling

Bone contains bone remodeling units (BRUs) at discrete locations and at different developmental stages. The function and arrangement of these small subunits, which constantly "turn over" bone matrix constituents and mineral, create the basis for the changes in bone mass and structure observed with increasing age and in metabolic bone disease.

Every remodeling cycle is initiated by the activation of osteoclastic precursors to become multinucleated osteoclasts and start osteoclastic bone resorption. After resorption is terminated, the area is invaded by preosteoblasts that differentiate into osteoblasts, which form new matrix that subsequently becomes mineralized during continued osteoblastic bone formation. Bone remodeling is therefore often described as an activation-resorption-formation (A–R–F) sequence (Table 2). The remodeling period, i.e., the duration of the complete remodeling sequence, is commonly subdivided into an erosion period (EP) and a formation period (FP). In people with normal skeletal metabolism, the remodeling period is approximately 100 days in cortical bone and 200 days in cancellous bone.

THE REMODELING SEQUENCE IN CORTICAL BONE

In cortical bone, the resorption process (erosion period) lasts 30 days. During that period of time, a tunnel with a diameter of approximately 150 mm is created by osteoclastic and mononuclear resorption. The preosteoclastic phase lasts approximately 10 days, followed by a 15-day period of monocytic activity. After a 5-day period during which preosteoblasts arrive, the osteoblastic period of matrix formation ensues. Osteoblasts synthesize the matrix which, after about 15 to 20 days, undergoes mineralization. The formation period lasts about 90 days, during which new bone refills the tunnel (Fig. 2), leaving a mean wall thickness of approximately 40 mm to 60 mm and a central haversian canal with a diameter of approximately 30 mm.

THE REMODELING SEQUENCE IN CANCELLOUS BONE

In cancellous bone (Fig. 6), the erosion period lasts about 43 days and can be subdivided into a 7-day period of osteoclastic resorption and a 36-day period of mononuclear resorption during which a final erosion depth of approximately 60 mm is reached. Preosteoblasts migrate into the resorption cavity for 7 days before matrix formation starts. During this time, these preosteoblasts differentiate into osteoblasts. Matrix formation takes place for 15 days before signs of mineralization are detectable; this period between matrix formation and the initiation of mineralization is also called the initial mineralization lag time. The resorption cavity is filled with new bone to a final wall thickness of approximately 40 mm to 60 mm over a total period of about 145 days. Figure 7 illustrates this remodeling sequence in bone biopsy sections from cancellous bone.

The majority of bone formation in cancellous bone is coupled to the preceding bone resorption. However, under certain conditions (e.g., primary growth, Paget's disease of bone, fluoride therapy), *de novo* bone formation may occur on quiescent surfaces. In these instances, the initial bone formed will have a woven structure.

TABLE 2. *The A-R-F sequence of bone remodeling*

ACTIVATION	Activation of osteoclastic precursors.
RESORPTION	Initial resorption by osteoclasts.
	Later resorption by mononuclear cells.
FORMATION	Termination of resorption and invasion of resorption cavities by preosteoblasts.
	Differentiation of preosteoblasts into osteoblasts.
	Formation of new bone matrix and subsequent mineralization by osteoblasts.

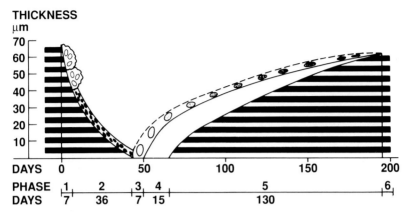

FIG. 6. The normal cancellous bone remodeling sequence, calculated from histomorphometric analysis of bone biopsy samples obtained from young individuals. Note the balance between the erosion depth and the mean wall thickness. Five different phases can be distinguished over time: osteoclastic resorption (**1**), mononuclear resorption (**2**), preosteoblastic migration and differentiation into osteoblasts (**3**), osteoblastic matrix (osteoid) formation (**4**), and mineralization (**5**). The end product of remodeling in cancellous bone is the completed cancellous bone structural unit (BSU) (i.e., trabecular osteon, wall or "packet" of bone) (**6**). Adapted from Eriksen *et al.* (59).

ACTIVATION FREQUENCY

The amount of bone remodeled per unit of time at the tissue level depends not only on osteoblastic and osteoclastic activity at each BRU site but also on the number of active remodeling sites per unit of bone volume. The rate at which BRUs are formed is called the activation frequency.

Although mean erosion depth and mean wall thickness may only vary by 10% to 20% in different diseases, activation frequency may vary by 50% to 100%. Thus, in most diseases, activation frequency is the most important regulator of bone turnover and changes in bone mass (3,6).

THE QUANTUM CONCEPT OF BONE REMODELING

According to the quantum concept of Frost (1,6), changes in bone mass are caused by an imbalance between the amount of bone resorbed by osteoclasts and the amount of bone formed by

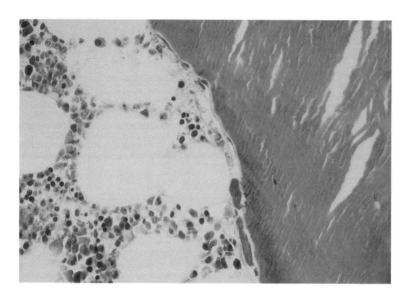

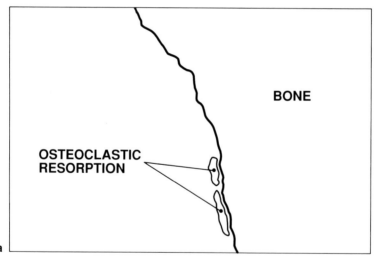

FIG. 7. Micrographs of the different phases of the remodeling sequence in cancellous bone as seen in a bone biopsy section. The phases of osteoclastic and mononuclear resorption (**a**), preosteoblasts (**b, p.17**), and osteoblastic matrix (osteoid) formation (**c, p.18**) are shown. The completed bone structural unit (BSU, trabecular osteon) covered by lining cells is shown in partially polarized light to demonstrate the lamellar characteristics of the final wall or "packet" of bone (**d, p.19**). **a,b**, Masson-Trichrome, x 500; **c**, Goldner-Trichrome, x 200; **d**, Masson-Trichrome, x 500.

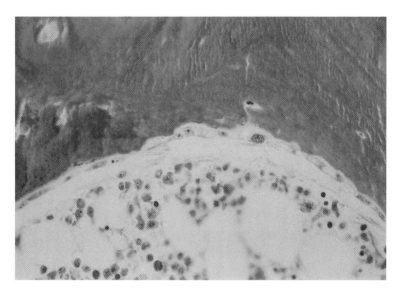

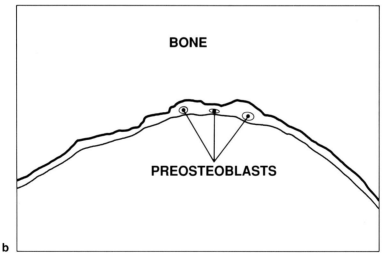

FIG. 7. Continued.

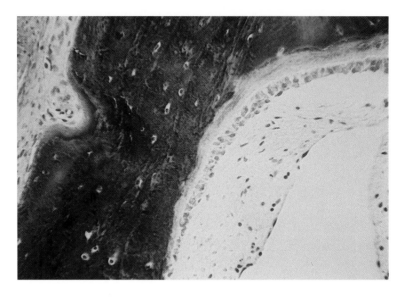

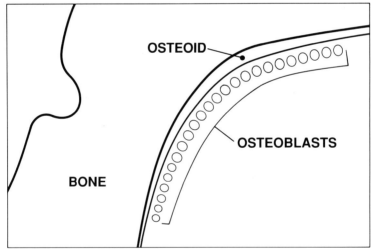

FIG. 7. Continued.

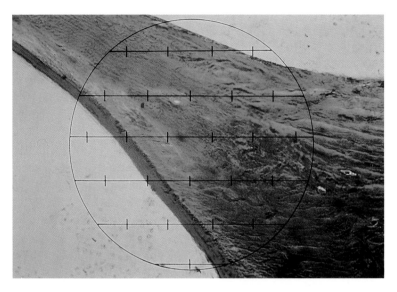

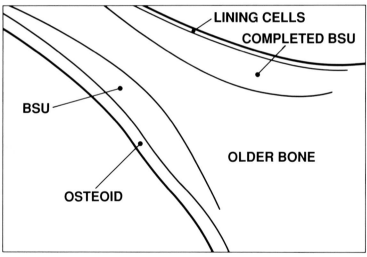

FIG. 7. Continued.

osteoblasts at each individual BRU site. After the termination of bone resorption, bone formation is initiated in the resorption cavity through "coupling" Under normal circumstances, the coupling process ensures that the amount of bone removed is deposited again during the subsequent formation phase. The term coupling denotes a temporal sequence of events, whereas the term "imbalance" is used to describe circumstances in which the resorption cavities either are incompletely refilled (if resorption exceeds formation) or are overfilled (if formation exceeds resorption) (3,6). Each BRU represents a "quantum" of bone remodeling activity. These quantal activities may be moderated by disease or therapy by changing the intrinsic activities, such as erosion depth or wall thickness. The overall skeletal response to remodeling reflects the summation of these quantal events over time.

The mechanical stimulation of bone cells appears to be important to the coupling process. Immobilization (e.g., during bed rest or the weightlessness of space flight) leads to a pronounced negative bone balance as a result of the "uncoupling" of resorption and formation. In the weight-bearing skeleton, trabeculae lacking connections to other trabeculae may also show signs of this uncoupling of the resorptive and formative activities (7).

SUMMARY

Bone remodeling is initiated by the recruitment of *osteoclasts* and subsequent bone *resorption*, which is then followed by the recruitment of *osteoblasts* and subsequent *formation* of bone matrix and its mineralization.

In normal bone, the duration of the *remodeling period* ranges from 100 days in cortical bone to 200 days in cancellous bone.

Activation frequency is the frequency at which new bone remodeling units (BRUs) are activated.

Coupling describes the temporal sequence of events that ensures that osteoclastic resorption is followed by osteoblastic formation at any given bone remodeling unit (BRU) site.

The term *"imbalance"* describes the circumstances in which resorption cavities (lacunae) either are incompletely refilled or are overfilled.

CHAPTER FOUR

Bone Remodeling and Changes in Bone Mass

REVERSIBLE CHANGES IN BONE MASS

A reversible loss of bone may occur if the number of resorption cavities suddenly increases, leading to an expansion of the remodeling space. Because of the activation-resorption-formation sequence, this will occur before bone formation increases and thus lead to a decrease in trabecular bone mass. However, once bone formation has proceeded, bone mass will stabilize at a new lower level, provided no net deficit exists between resorption and formation at the individual bone remodeling unit (BRU) level. In contrast, a reduction of the remodeling space will occur if the activation frequency decreases (e.g., as a result of estrogen therapy, bisphosphonate therapy, or a reduction in thyroid hormone status), leading to an increase in bone density. Several studies have demonstrated that changes in remodeling space may be responsible for changes of 5% to 15% in bone mass (8,9).

In cortical bone, increased remodeling activity (such as that seen in hyperthyroidism or primary hyperparathyroidism) leads to increased cortical porosity and apparent loss of bone mass. Figure 8a shows how a decrease in activation frequency affects the porosity of cortical bone. Changes in cortical porosity will be especially obvious if bone mass measurements are performed at skeletal sites that are predominantly cortical bone (e.g., the forearm) (Fig. 9).

In cancellous bone, decreased bone turnover will also decrease the number of resorption cavities per unit volume of bone and thus decrease its porosity (Fig. 8b). An increase in turnover will have the

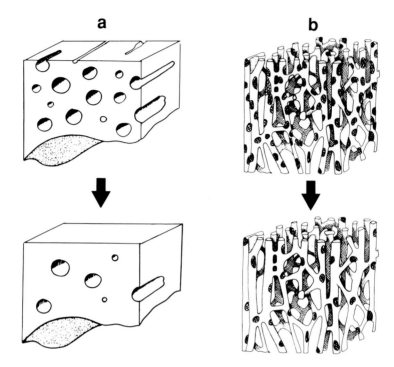

FIG. 8. Effect of activation frequency on bone porosity. In cortical bone (**a**), remodeling sites (osteons) are depicted as tunnels within the bone; in cancellous bone (**b**), they are depicted as pits on the surfaces of the trabeculae. In both types of bone, a decrease in activation frequency leads to fewer remodeling sites at steady state with a subsequent decrease in porosity.

opposite effect, and, as will be discussed, the architectural impact of a higher rate of turnover in combination with increased erosion depth may be important in leading to trabecular loss.

IRREVERSIBLE CHANGES IN BONE MASS

In cortical bone, irreversible bone loss may be caused by excessive endosteal resorption (Fig. 10) or increased haversian canal diameter leading to increased porosity of the cortex (12).

In cancellous bone, irreversible bone loss may occur as a result of a negative balance per remodeling cycle at each BRU site, thus resulting in trabecular thinning or perforative resorption and the loss of trabecular elements (Fig. 10). Trabecular perforations constitute the main mecha-

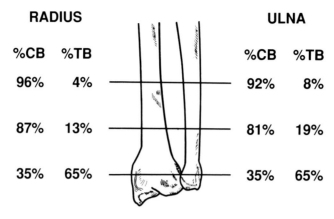

FIG. 9. Percentage of cortical bone (CB) and trabecular bone (TB) at different sites in the forearm. From Melsen *et al.* (10).

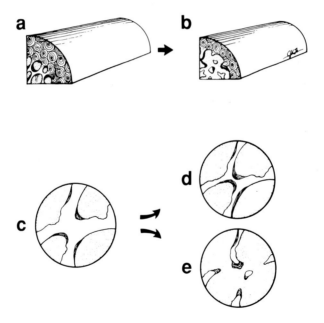

FIG. 10. Irreversible bone loss in cortical and cancellous bone. A remodeling imbalance favoring endosteal resorption (**a**) leads to cortical thinning (**b**). Resorption without adequate formation (**c**) leads to trabecular thinning (**d**) and perforation (**e**) in cancellous bone. Adapted from Eriksen *et al.* (11).

nism by which cancellous bone is irreversibly lost and are caused by an inequality between trabecular thickness and erosion depth (6,13). A perforation occurs either when one resorptive cavity penetrates completely through the trabeculum from one side or when two cavities meet midway

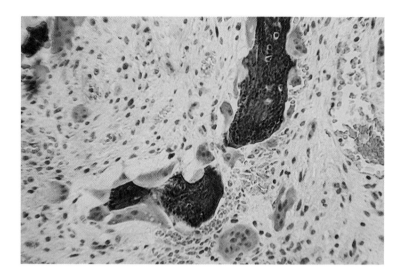

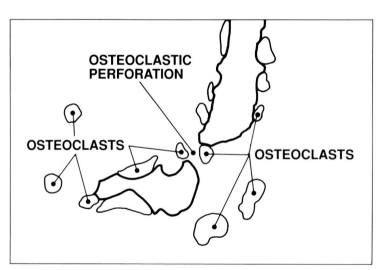

FIG. 11. Osteoclastic perforation of a trabeculum, as seen in biopsy section studied with light microscopy. Goldner-Trichrome, x 200.

through the trabeculum (Fig.10) (6). The statistical probability of a perforation depends on the activation frequency, the depth of the resorptive cavities, and the thickness of trabeculae (3,6). Each time a trabeculum is perforated, a certain amount of trabecular bone is irreversibly lost. Gradually, the plates forming the trabecular "honeycomb" pattern are converted into a lattice of bars and rods, some of which in turn may be transected or completely removed through further resorptive activity (Fig. 11). This sequence of events has been confirmed by scanning electron microscopy (14,15) and leads directly to the loss of overall architectural continuity and strength in cancellous bone (Fig. 12, see pages 26–28).

Increased bone turnover by itself may also lead to a negative bone balance and net bone loss. This has been demonstrated by calcium kinetic and histomorphometric methods and occurs in osteoporosis. For example, in a study of 58 patients with osteoporosis, Eriksen *et al.* (16) found a more negative BRU balance with increased turnover. These findings probably reflect a combination of changes that include an increased risk of trabecular perforations by virtue of a greater number of resorptive events on trabecular bone.

SUMMARY

Reversible bone loss is caused primarily by changes in the rate of bone turnover (activation frequency), leading to an increased porosity of *cortical bone* and an increased number of resorption cavities in *cancellous bone.*

Irreversible bone loss in cortical bone is caused primarily by increased *endosteal resorption.*

Irreversible bone loss in cancellous bone is caused primarily by negative bone balance at the BRU level and subsequent *trabecular perforations*, leading to disintegration of the trabecular network.

The *risk of trabecular perforations* increases with increasing erosion depth, increasing activation frequency, and decreasing trabecular integrity (trabecular thinning).

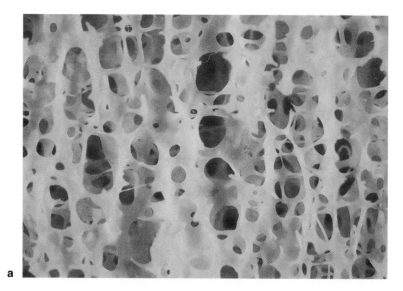

a

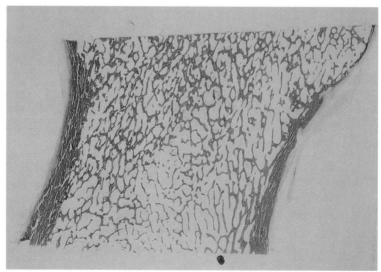

b

FIG. 12. Cancellous bone obtained from vertebrae and femoral necks, respectively, of normal (**a,b**), osteoporotic (**c,d**), and severely osteoporotic subjects (**e,f**). Note the loss of trabecular continuity due to resorptive perforations in the severely osteoporotic subject. **b,d,f**, Masson-Trichrome, x 25.

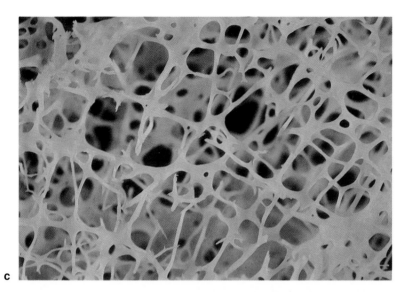

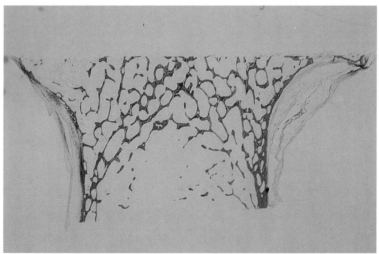

FIG. 12. Continued.

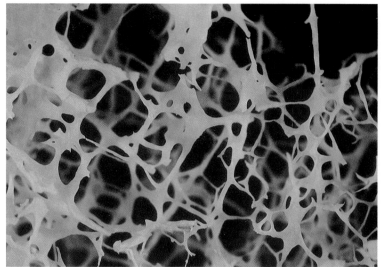

e

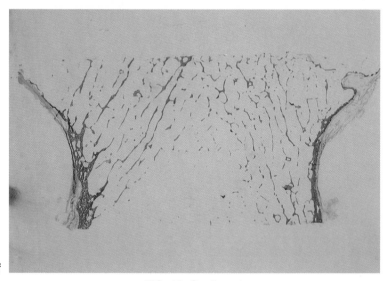

f

FIG. 12. Continued.

Bone Remodeling and Bone Mass Measurements

The use of photon absorptiometry has emerged as a sensitive and convenient method for assessing bone mass. The interpretation of bone mass data, however, relies heavily on an understanding of bone remodeling. As previously mentioned, cortical and cancellous bone exhibit pronounced differences in architecture, remodeling activity, and mechanisms of bone loss. These differences may lead to different alterations in bone density in different areas of the skeleton, depending on the proportions of cortical and cancellous bone (17).

Changes in remodeling activity lead to changes in porosity and absolute bone mass but also affect the mean age of bone. Because older bone is more heavily mineralized than younger bone, changes in the mean age of bone, with the slow accumulation of additional mineral, introduce an extra variable (8,9). Mathematical modeling based on available histomorphometric data suggests that, in extreme cases, bone mass measurements may deviate by as much as 40% from "true" bone mass, as defined by the volume of calcified bone. More commonly, however, the deviation amounts to 5% to 15%.

Three different patterns of changes in bone mass are seen when analyzing the effects of various treatments affecting bone metabolism. The first pattern (Fig. 13a) shows a steady increase in bone mass continuing during the treatment period with no plateau reached. It may be explained by a slow rise to steady state or by an anabolic effect, leading to pronounced increases in bone remodel-

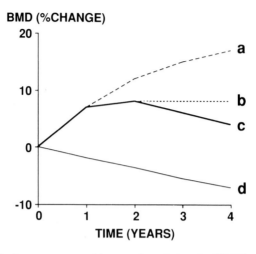

FIG. 13. Typical appearance of bone mineral density (BMD) curves representative of responses to different types of treatment. Treatment with anabolic agents that greatly increase bone formation leads to continued gains in bone mass (**a**). Treatment with agents that decrease bone turnover can lead to initial increases in bone mass with subsequent plateau (**b**) or loss (age-dependent) (**c**) compared with persistent bone loss in the untreated state (**d**). Adapted from Eriksen *et al.* (18).

ing unit (BRU) balance. This pattern has only been reported to occur with agents that stimulate bone formation, such as fluoride (19) and, to a lesser degree, combination therapy with parathyroid hormone and 1,25-dihydroxyvitamin D_3 (20).

A second pattern (Fig. 13b) is exhibited in patients treated with bisphosphonate therapy and occurs in some studies of estrogen/progestin therapy. Initial gains of 5% to 10% in bone mass are maintained throughout treatment (21,22). Provided the measurement device is stable over time and the mean age of bone does not change, this pattern can only be explained by a modest anabolic effect offsetting age-dependent bone loss.

A third pattern (Fig. 13c) is typified by a 5% to 10% increase in bone mass, usually observed after 1 year of intervention, after which, bone mass levels off and ultimately starts to decrease. The initial increase is explained by a decrease in bone turnover, with a contraction of the remodeling space, leading to an increase in bone mass. After 2-3 years of intervention, however, age-dependent bone loss begins to offset the initial gain, and bone mass may again decrease. This pattern has been reported in some studies of bone mass changes after therapy with estrogen/progestin (23) or calcitonin (24); however, in the case of calcitonin, the loss of bone mass after 2 years may relate to a loss of drug efficacy, rather than to opposing mechanisms of bone loss, such as trabecular loss.

Agents that decrease turnover, such as bisphosphonates, estrogen/progestin, and calcitonin, are commonly described as antiresorptive. However, their action may reflect two effects: a decrease in resorption depth (a true antiresorptive effect) and an inhibition of the initiation of new remodeling units (an antiactivation effect). Both of these effects may work in concert to increase bone mass and decrease irreversible bone loss, as discussed earlier. Estrogen inhibits bone resorption, mediated by a reduction in the activation frequency of new bone remodeling cycles, but has no effect on the depth of resorption cavities; it is the decrease in the number of these cavities (Fig. 8b) that translates into increased bone mass. Calcitonin also acts through inhibition of bone resorption, but its effects on resorption depth and activation are unknown. Only the bisphosphonates have been shown to exhibit both antiresorptive and antiactivation effects.

SUMMARY

Measurements of bone mass are affected by the *turnover state* of the skeleton.

Therapies that stimulate bone formation (e.g., fluoride, parathyroid hormone/1,25-dihydroxyvitamin D_3) can lead to progressive increases in bone mass.

Antiresorptive therapies (e.g., estrogen/progestin, calcitonin, bisphosphonates) can lead to initial increases in bone mass, which then levels off and either is maintained or decreases.

CHAPTER SIX

Bone Histology and Histomorphometry

Bone histology is the study of bone by light microscopy. It provides qualitative information, including the overall structure and distribution of bone components.

Bone histomorphometry includes the measurement of morphologic components, such as osteoid thickness and wall thickness. These are *static* variables that are measured directly. Histomorphometry can also estimate *kinetic* variables through the use of fluorescent labels, administered at timed intervals, that integrate into forming bone. The distance between such labels provides information about the rate of bone formation and, by derivation, about other bone metabolic processes as well. Finally, newer *reconstructive* techniques provide insight into the magnitude and rate of ongoing processes in bone without including contributions from preexisting bone elements that might otherwise bias the kinetic assessment.

THE BASIS FOR HISTOMORPHOMETRIC EVALUATION

A unique feature of bone is that both past and current cellular events are represented in a bone biopsy sample. Bone remodeling leaves "traces" that can be quantitated by microscopic and stereologic analysis; these "traces" may represent events that occurred several years ago. The incorporation of tetracycline labels (Fig. 14) into bone as time markers(1) also permits the dynamic description of current remodeling activity. These characteristics form the basis for the calculation of the rates of activity of the different cell types (1,3).

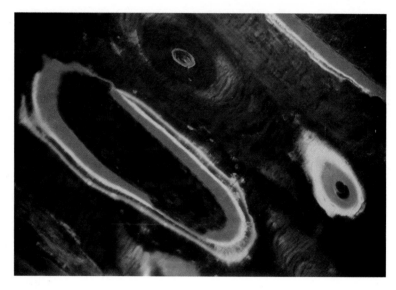

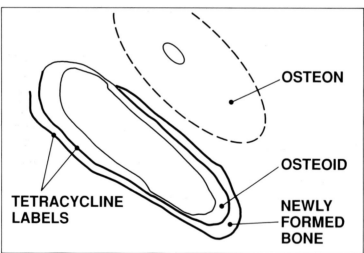

FIG. 14. Tetracycline double labels in cortical bone as seen in fluorescence microscopy. Note the distance between the two labels. The thickness of bone between the two labels has been formed over a period of 10 days. This thickness divided by the labeling interval (10 days) yields the mineral appositional rate (MAR). Villanueva, x 500.

Bone densitometry, assays of biochemical markers in the serum, and calcium kinetics studies can only yield data on tissue- or organ-level activity, which therefore reflect individual cell activity as well as cell number. Quantitative bone histology is the only method by which alterations in cellular activity can be separated from changes in cell number.

INDICATIONS FOR BONE BIOPSY

Apart from the clear utility of bone histomorphometry in bone research and clinical therapeutics, bone histomorphometric methods can also be useful in clinical practice. Table 3 describes several indications for bone biopsy in the clinical setting. In general, patients with poor responses to therapy may benefit from a more detailed analysis of bone histology and histomorphometry.

BONE BIOPSY PROCEDURES AND SAMPLE PREPARATION TECHNIQUES

The sequence of the histomorphometric method is outlined in Table 4. Before the bone biopsy procedure, the patient receives two separate doses of a tetracycline derivative at a 10- to 14-day interval. The biopsy procedure itself is safe and can be performed under a local anesthetic. Bone biopsy samples are most frequently obtained from the anterior ilium by drilling out a transcortical cylinder with a diameter of 0.6 cm to 0.8 cm; this sample size provides adequate material for most histomorphometric analyses. The biopsy core is then fixed in either ethanol or formalin.

TABLE 3. *Indications for bone biopsy in the clinical setting*

- Suspected osteomalacia
- Diagnostic classification of renal osteodystrophy
- Osteopenia in young individuals (younger than 50 years of age)
- Osteopenia in individuals with abnormal calcium metabolism
- Hereditary childhood bone diseases that present problems in terms of classification
- Evaluation of treatment in certain diseases (e.g., osteomalacia, hypophosphatasia)

TABLE 4. *Sequence of histomorphometric method*

- Administration of two separate doses of tetracycline derivative at a 10- to 14-day interval before biopsy procedure.
- Biopsy of transiliac bone.
- Fixation of biopsy sample in ethanol or formalin.
- Embedding of sample in hard plastic.
- Sectioning of sample on heavy-duty microtome.
- Staining (e.g., Goldner-Trichrome, Masson-Trichrome, Toluidine Blue, Villanueva) or no staining (for analysis of tetracycline labeling) of sec tion, as appropriate.
- Qualitative and quantitative analysis of sections with light, polarized light, and fluorescence microscopy; optical grid systems; and computerized digitizing devices.

Bone histomorphometric analysis requires the use of sections of undecalcified bone. Before sectioning, the bone biopsy sample must be embedded in a hard plastic and sectioned with a special heavy-duty microtome. The sections are then left unstained (for analysis of tetracycline labeling) or suitably stained to provide sufficient cellular detail and separation of osteoid from mineralized bone. The Villanueva staining method permits simultaneous visualization and analysis of tetracycline labels, osteoid, and mineralized bone (Fig. 14). Quantitative microscopic analysis is performed with light, polarized light, and fluorescence microscopy; optical grid systems (to ensure proper random positioning); and computerized digitizing devices. A digitizing tablet is employed with the grid system to quantitate the size (width, thickness, and depth) and the number of structures (e.g., osteoid, final wall, and resorption cavity) in cortical (Fig. 15a) and cancellous (Fig. 15b) bone. In this way, measurements can be obtained without bias.

It is important to properly perform the bone biopsy procedure and prepare the bone samples and sections. The use of a sample that is too small or that has been damaged during biopsy may substantially reduce the amount and quality of the data obtained. Table 5 lists the criteria for good quality biopsy samples and sections.

TABLE 5. *Criteria for good quality bone biopsy samples and sections*

Sample
  Both cortices present and intact.
  Sample uncompressed and untwisted.
  Adequate material for complete analysis.

Section
  Trabecular structure intact (e.g., no cracks or fractures).
  Marrow closely aligned with trabecular surfaces.
  Staining appropriate (no over - or understaining).
  Tetracycline labels intact (not faded or washed out).

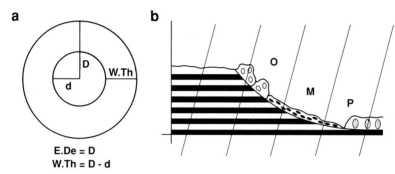

FIG. 15. Assessment of erosion depth and wall thickness in cortical bone (**a**) and erosion depth in cancellous bone (**b**). In cortical bone, erosion depth and wall thickness are calculated from the outer and inner diameters (D and d, respectively) of the "haversian system" (cortical osteon). Erosion depth (E.De) is described by D, whereas wall thickness (W.Th) is described by the difference between the two diameters (D – d). In cancellous bone, erosion depth is based on the number of lamellae eroded under the three different cell types that can be distinguished in resorption cavities: osteoclasts (O), mononuclear cells (M), and preosteoblasts (P). The final erosion depth is described by the mean number of lamellae at measuring sites containing preosteoblasts. The mean depths under osteoclasts and mononuclear cells can be used for reconstruction of the total erosion sequence. Adapted from Eriksen *et al.* (25).

SUMMARY

Bone *biopsy samples* reflect both *past and current bone cellular events.*

The use of *tetracycline double labels* permits the incorporation of a time marker into bone.

Bone biopsy samples are most frequently obtained from the *anterior ilium.*

Bone histomorphometric analysis requires the use of *sections of undecalcified bone.*

The biopsy samples must be embedded in a *hard plastic* before sectioning with a *heavy-duty microtome.*

Unstained or Villanueva-stained bone biopsy sections are used for the analysis of *tetracycline labeling.*

For other analyses, *suitable stains* are used to provide sufficient cellular detail and separation of osteoid from mineralized bone in the biopsy sections.

Histomorphometric analysis is performed with *light, polarized light, and fluorescence microscopy; optical grid systems; and computerized digitizing devices.*

CHAPTER SEVEN

Histomorphometric Indices

PRIMARY AND SECONDARY HISTOMORPHOMETRIC INDICES

There are many histomorphometric indices (3,26,27), some of which are of greater utility to the clinician than others. Described here are those that are the most relevant in clinical practice. A flow chart for the histomorphometric analysis of bone biopsy samples is shown in Table 6.

Primary histomorphometric indices are those that are measured directly on the histologic section. They include the following.

1. *Cell number*, i.e., the enumeration of cell profiles in a section (e.g., the number of osteoblasts or osteoclasts per millimeter of suface).

2. *Surface estimates*, i.e., the measurement of the extent of surface covered with a structure (e.g., the percent osteoid surface).

3. *Structure widths*, i.e., the measurement of the width of a struc ture (e.g., osteoid thickness or wall width or thickness).

4. *Erosion depth*, i.e., the depth of the resorption cavity, as mea sured in lamellae from the surface.

5. *Interlabel width*, i.e., the measurement of the distance between tetracycline double labels, as used in the calculation of mineral appositional rate.

Secondary (derived) histomorphometric indices are calculated from the primary indices and include erosion (resorption) period and formation period, erosion (resorption) and formation rates, mineralization lag time, and activation frequency. From these derived indices, a

TABLE 6. *Flow chart for histomorphometric analyses of bone biopsy samples*

1. Measurement of surface-related indices (by light microscopy).
   Cell number (as number of osteoblasts [N.Ob] and osteoclasts [N.Oc])
   Erosion surface as a fraction of bone surface (ES/BS)
   Osteoid surface as a fraction of bone surface (OS/BS)
   Active erosion surface (erosion surface covered by osteoclasts and mononuclear cells) (a.ES)
   Surface-to-volume ratio (BS/BV)

2. Measurement of structure thickness and erosion depth (by light microscopy and polarized light microscopy).
   Erosion depth (E.De)
   Wall thickness (W.Th)
   Osteoid thickness (O.Th)

3. Measurement of tetracycline labels (by fluorescence microscopy) and calculation of tetracycline-based surface indices.
   Labeled surface (LS) (or mineralizing surface [MS])
   Labeled surface as a fraction of bone surface (LS/BS)
   Mineral appositional rate (MAR) = distance between labels/labeling period

4. Calculation of derived indices based on surface indices and structure thickness.
   Adjusted appositional rate (Aj.AR) = MAR x (LS/OS)
   Formation period (FP) = life span of osteoid surface = W.Th/Aj.AR
   Erosion period (EP) = life span of erosion surface = FP x (ES/OS)
   Active erosion period (a.EP) = life span of osteoclasts and mononuclear cells = FP x (a.Es/OS)
   Erosion rate (ER) = E.De/a.EP
   Mineralization lag time (Mlt) = O.Th/Aj.AR
   Volume-referent bone resorption rate (BRs.R/BV)= a.ES x ER x (BS/BV)
   Volume-referent bone formation rate (BFR/BV)= MS x MAR x (BS/BV)
   Activation frequency (Ac.f) = (FP x [BS/OS]) $^{-1}$ = (EP + FP + QP) $^{-1}$

5. Reconstruction of the remodeling sequence.

---

full reconstruction of the remodeling sequence can also be performed.

One important prerequisite for the calculation of derived indices is the existence of "steady state," i.e., the state in which the activation frequency (birth rate) of new resorption cavities is equal to the activation frequency of new formation sites. If bone biopsies are performed too early after a change in disease state or after the initiation of treatment, only bone resorption will have been affected, while bone formation will still be proceeding at previous rates. In these non-steady-state conditions, the calculation of functional periods (e.g., erosion period, formation perioid) may yield false results.

CELL NUMBER

Obtaining the correct estimates of cell number in a section is difficult and involves time-consuming advanced stereologic techniques. The major problem is determining whether two neighboring cross-sectional profiles belong to the same cell or to two different cells. The only unbiased method for enumeration of these cross-sectional cell profiles involves the use of dissector techniques (i.e., the study of two sections separated by a given small distance, e.g., 10 μm) (28). The dissector can be either physical (i.e., two sections taken with the given separation) or optical (i.e., two sections viewed with confocal microscopy). The two sections are then studied side by side, and the differences in profile shapes are counted.

The identification of osteoblasts and osteoclasts by purely morphologic criteria is usually straightforward, but histochemical staining (e.g., alkaline phosphatase for osteoblasts and tartrate-resistant phosphatase for osteoclasts) may be helpful.

SURFACE ESTIMATES

Surface estimates reflect the extent of surface covered by osteoid or tetracycline labels or undergoing resorption. They are most often given as a fraction of the total bone surface (e.g., osteoid-covered surface [OS/BS], labeled surface [LS/BS], and erosion surface [ES/BS]) and provide the basis for the calculation of a wide variety of derived histomorphometric indices. An important surface-based estimate is the ratio between bone surface and the volume of trabecular bone (BS/BV), which gives the bone surface area within a given volume of bone as estimated from measurements of both the perimeter and the area of the trabecular structures.

Surface estimates have often been misinterpreted. For example, increases in the extent of eroded surface have been taken as a sign of increased resorptive activity. However, this may be misleading because the extent of eroded surface depends on two factors (Fig. 16): the life span of the resorption cavity and the birth rate of new cavities. This may be expressed by the simple formula below.

Extent of surface = activation frequency x life span of surface

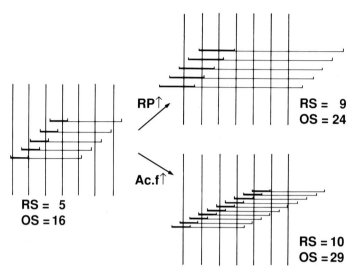

FIG. 16. The effects of changes in activation frequency (birth rate of new remodeling cycles) and duration of remodeling periods on the extent of bone surface covered by resorptive surfaces (RS) or formative (osteoid-covered) surfaces (OS). Each single remodeling cycle with its individual erosion and formation periods is represented by one step on the classic ladder diagram originally proposed by Frost (1). This diagram shows remodeling cycles separated in both time and space. A doubling of the remodeling period (RP) is shown as a doubling of the length of each ladder and its individual erosion and formation periods without any change in the total number of ladders. A doubling of the activation frequency (Ac.f) is shown as a doubling of the number of ladders, without any change in the length of the individual ladders. When counting intersections between grid lines (vertical lines) and erosion or formation sites, both changes in remodeling will cause the same increase in the number of intersections and surface estimates (RS and OS) as compared with the basal situation. From Eriksen *et al.*(47).

Thus, an increased duration of the resorptive process, which may be a sign of reduced resorptive activity, may actually result in increased resorption surface. The same considerations hold for all other surface estimates. The determination of surface estimates should therefore only be considered an intermediate step necessary for the calculation of relevant derived indices.

EROSION AND FORMATION PERIODS

With the previously described formula for surface extent, it is possible to calculate the life span or functional periods of the formative and resorptive cells by combining surface estimates and tetracycline-label-based indices. These formulas (Table 6) are based on the calculation of the formation period (FP) and the use of this index to calculate the erosion period (EP), i.e., the life span of the erosion surface.

ACTIVATION FREQUENCY

In cortical bone, activation frequency (Ac.f) is relatively easy to determine because the number of bone remodeling units (BRUs) per unit volume of bone can be counted. In cancellous (trabecular) bone, however, another approach must be employed (2,29). The duration of the remodeling cycle in cancellous bone is the sum of the resorption and formation periods. The end of the formation period (FP) is followed by a long quiescent period (QP), during which no remodeling activity occurs on the surface. In cancellous bone, the sum of the resorptive, formative, and quiescent periods represents the interval from the initiation of one remodeling cycle to the initiation of the next at the same point on the trabecular surface. Thus, activation frequency, or the rate at which new remodeling cycles are initiated, is the reciprocal of this total period and is calculated by the following equation.

$$\text{Ac.f (time}^{-1}) = (EP + FP + QP)^{-1} \text{ or } (FP \times [BS/OS])^{-1}$$

TISSUE-LEVEL VOLUME-REFERENT INDICES

Bone turnover is best described in terms of the *volume* of bone resorbed and formed. Volume-referent indices describing tissue-level bone resorption (BRs.R/BV) and tissue-level bone formation (BFR/BV) are easily calculated based on the surface estimates (2,30). The calculations (shown subsequently) are based on the surface measurement (active erosion surface or eroded surface covered by osteoclasts [a.ES] or mineralizing surface [MS]), the rate of activity at the given surface (erosion rate [ER] or mineral appositional rate [MAR]), and a conversion factor transforming the two-dimensional surface-based index for resorption or formation into a three-dimensional index (BS/BV, which is the surface-to-volume ratio or the area of surface per unit volume).

$$BRs.R/BV = a.ES \times ER \times (BS/BV)$$

$$BFR/BV = MS \times MAR \times (BS/BV)$$

The volume-referent bone balance (Dt.BV/BV) is the difference between the volume-referent indices of formation and resorption.

$$Dt.BV/BV = BFR/BV - BRs.R/BV$$

These indices correlate significantly with whole skeletal turnover, as assessed by calcium balance and calcium kinetic studies (30,31).

RECONSTRUCTION OF THE REMODELING SEQUENCE

A convenient way to represent most of the important indices discussed is in the form of a curve showing changes in the remodeling site over time. As shown in Fig. 17, cellular activity, erosion depth, osteoid thickness, and mineralized matrix can be displayed as a function of time. This type of presentation provides a perspective on the duration of the erosion and formation periods and shows directly any net imbalance at the BRU level at the end of the remodeling period.

KEY INDICES OF BONE REMODELING
AND BONE BALANCE

The pertinent indices for describing bone remodeling are listed in Table 7. The effects of alterations in the key histomorphometric indices of erosion depth, wall thickness, and activation frequency on trabecular thickness, extent of trabecular perforations, and cortical characteristics are shown in Table 8.

Changes in bone mass depend on two main factors: the balance between resorption and formation at the BRU level and the number of active remodeling sites. Bone balance at each remodeling site is reflected in the difference between the depth of the resorption cavity (erosion depth) and the thickness of bone at the completed remodel-

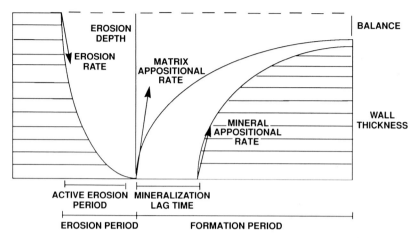

FIG. 17. Key indices of bone remodeling as calculated from remodeling curves. This graphic reconstruction of the remodeling sequence yields information on the rates of activity of the different cell populations (erosion and formation rates, i.e., the rates of matrix and mineral apposition), the duration of erosion and formation periods, and the final result of cellular activity through these periods (i.e., final erosion depth and wall thickness). The vertical distance between matrix and mineral appositional rate curves represents the osteoid thickness of any time point. The mineralization lag time is described by the horizontal distance between these matrix and mineral growth curves. The difference between erosion depth and wall thickness describes the balance at the level of individual bone remodeling units (BRUs). Adapted from Eriksen *et al.* (18).

ing site (wall thickness). The number of active remodeling sites at a given time is reflected in the activation frequency (the frequency at which new remodeling sites are activated in the cortex or on the trabecular surface).

The total resorptive activity can also be calculated per unit of bone tissue as the volume of bone removed per unit of time. Formative activity can similarly be calculated as the volume of bone formed per unit of time. Bone balance is then calculated as the difference between "volume-referent" resorption and formation rates. These indices reflect the activity at each remodeling site multiplied by the activation frequency.

In cortical bone, the erosion depth is equivalent to the cross-sectional radius of the osteon (12,32). The mean wall thickness is equivalent to the distance from the haversian canal to the osteon perimeter

TABLE 7. *Pertinent indices for the description of bone remodeling*

Descriptor	Index	Abbreviation
Resorption	Erosion depth	E.De
	Erosion rate,bone remodeling unit (BRU) level	ER
	Bone resorption rate, volume-referent	BRs.R/BV
Formation	Mean wall thickness	W.Th
	Osteoid thickness	O.Th
	Mineral appositional rate	MAR
	Bone formation rate, volume-referent	BFR/BV
	Mineralization lag time	Mlt
Balance	Bone balance, BRU level = mean W.Th − E.De	Dt.BRU
	Bone balance, volume-referent = BFR/BV − BRs.R/BV)	Dt.BV/BV
Tissue-level Turnover	Activation frequency	Ac.f

and is easily calculated as D− d, where D is the cross-sectional radius of the osteon and d is the cross-sectional radius of the haversian canal (Fig.15a). A negative balance between resorption and formation will be reflected in an increased diameter of the haversian canal relative to the total diameter of the osteon. No positive balance can be achieved during cortical remodeling because even neutral balance would lead to complete filling of the haversian canal.

In cancellous bone, the depth of a resorption cavity (erosion depth) is measured with polarized light microscopy by counting the number of lamellae eroded in the completed cavity (Fig.15b) (25). In normal bone, these lamellae have a constant thickness of 3.2 μm. This thickness exhibits low interindividual variance and also remains constant in most metabolic bone diseases. Other methods for assessment of erosion depth, including either computerized (33) or free-hand (28) reconstruction of the eroded surface, have been described.

The overall osteoblastic activity is reflected in the mean wall thickness, which is the thickness of the bone packet that replaces the bone previously resorbed (Fig. 17). The distance between the tetracycline double labels reflects the rate of bone formation (Fig. 14). When

TABLE 8. *Consequences of changes in key histomorphometric indices*

Index	Direction of change	Consequences
Erosion depth	↑	↓ trabecular thickness ↑ perforations ↓ cortical thickness
	↓	↑ trabecular thickness ↓ perforations ↑ cortical thickness
Wall thickness	↑	↑ trabecular thickness ↓ perforations ↑ cortical thickness
	↓	↓ trabecular thickness ↑ perforations ↓ cortical thickness
Activation frequency	↑	↑ perforations ↑ cortical porosity
	↓	↓ perforations ↓ cortical porosity

adjusted for the time between the administration of the labels, this distance represents the mineral appositional rate, an important index in bone kinetics.

REGIONAL ACCELERATORY PHENOMENON

When bone biopsy samples are obtained from skeletal sites previously subjected to biopsy or injury (e.g., fracture), processes associated with healing or repair may result in falsely elevated kinetic turnover indices (i.e., those describing frequency and rates) and biased resorption and formation indices that do not reflect the status of bone remodeling in the rest of the skeleton. Frost (34,35) originally proposed the acronym RAP (regional acceleratory phenomenom) to describe this state. Because of the possible perturbation of data derived from sites undergoing or suspected to be undergoing RAP, repeat biopsies from the same skeletal site are not recommended unless they are separated by an extended period of time (several years).

SUMMARY

Primary histomorphometric indices are measured directly on the histologic section.

Secondary derived histomorphometric indices can provide biologically more meaningful information and are calculated from the primary indices.

The calculation of *functional periods* (e.g., erosion period or EP, formation period or FP) rely on the fact that the extent of a given surface is proportional to the life span of that surface.

Volume-referent estimates of resorption and formation rates can be calculated by the general formula *extent of surface x rate of activity x surface-to-volume ratio (or BS/BV).*

The *remodeling sequence* can be *reconstructed* from derived resorption indices and provides a graphic summary of the remodeling cycle.

Changes in bone mass depend on two main factors: the balance between resorption and formation and the number of active remodeling sites.

A *regional acceleratory phenomenom* (RAP) may occur at skeletal sites previously subjected to biopsy or injury; repeat biopsies at the same site may therefore yield data that do not reflect the status of bone remodeling in the rest of the skeleton.

CHAPTER EIGHT

Bone Structure and Bone Strength

Bone strength and fracture risk depend on bone structure (36,37). Between the ages of 20 and 80 years, a 60% to 65% decline in the compressive strength of the vertebral bodies occurs (38). There is no sex-related difference in the rate of decline, but overall, men display higher maximum load values than women as a result of the larger cross-sectional area of the vertebral bodies.

The compressive strength of vertebral bodies may be a good indicator of the risk of vertebral fracture but cannot be tested *in vivo*. In normal subjects, however, the average compressive strength of the vertebral bodies (or load, measured in Newtons) can be estimated from mechanical tests on iliac-crest bone cylinders (39).

One of the best descriptions of changes in the structure of cancellous bone is obtained by calculating marrow star volume (Fig. 18) (27). This index reflects the mean length of lines radiating from a given point in the marrow space until they intersect a trabeculum. The mean length of these lines will increase with an increasing number of perforations. Thus, an increase in the marrow star volume reflects an increase in the number of trabecular perforations. With increasing age, women display a larger increase in star volume than do men. This more pronounced disintegration of the trabecular network may therefore explain not only why women have a higher risk for osteoporotic vertebral fractures than men but also why women are more dependent on cortical bone for maintaining the biomechanical competence of vertebral bodies. As the trabecular architecture deteriorates, resistance to compressive fracture becomes more dependent on the cortical bone that serves as the circumferential vertebral "shell."

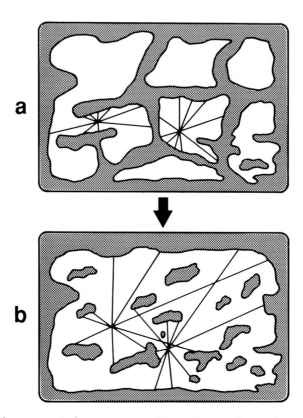

FIG. 18. Assessment of marrow star volume. From a given point within the marrow space, a number of lines radiate outward until they each intersect a trabeculum (**a**); the mean length of these lines is the marrow star volume. Loss of trabecular continuity through perforations (**b**) results in longer lines between the given point and the intersection with the remaining trabecular elements, i.e., an increase in marrow star volume.

CHAPTER NINE

Bone Remodeling in Metabolic Bone Disease

The bone loss seen in most metabolic bone diseases is explained by changes in remodeling and subsequent changes in bone balance at the bone remodeling unit (BRU) and tissue levels. Clearly, a complete study of a given metabolic bone disease should include an assessment of cortical bone remodeling, because cortical bone constitutes 80% of the skeleton. However, because of the slower turnover and different architecture of cortical bone, data on cortical remodeling are more difficult to obtain than those on cancellous bone remodeling. Some studies that combine data obtained from both cortical and cancellous bone have been published (40,41). Theoretically, these combined data should be better correlated to whole skeletal turnover; this correlation has been demonstrated experimentally (40). The characteristic changes in key histomorphometric indices in several important metabolic bone diseases are summarized in Table 9 and illustrated in Fig. 19.

OSTEOPOROSIS

Few studies have examined bone remodeling in osteoporotic subjects in comparison with that in age- and sex-matched normal subjects. Studies of the cortical osteon in osteoporotic subjects have not revealed any significant changes in osteon diameter or haversian canal diameter when compared with those in age-matched control subjects. Thus, in cortical bone, no negative balance was evident (12). The loss of cortical bone mass in osteoporosis may be

TABLE 9. *Bone remodeling of cortical and cancellous bone in different metabolic bone diseases, characterized by the following pertinent indices: mean wall thickness (W.Th), erosion depth (E.De), bone balance at the bone remodeling unit (BRU) level (Dt.BRU), mineralization lag time (Mlt), and activation frequency (Ac.f)*

Disease	W.Th	E.De	Dt.BRU	Mlt	Ac.f
Osteoporosis					
Cortical	→	→	o	→	→
Cancellous	↓	→	negative	→	(↑)
Osteomalacia					
Cortical	↓	↓	positive	↑	↑↓ [a]
Cancellous	?	?	?	↑	↑↓ [a]
Hyperthyroidism					
Cancellous	↓	→	negative	→	↑
Hypothyroidism					
Cortical	↑	↑	o	?	→
Cancellous	↑	↓	positive	↑	↓
Primary hyperparathyroidism					
Cortical	→	→	o	?	↑
Cancellous	↓	↓	o (negative)[b]	→	↑
Secondary hyperparathyroidism					
Cancellous	↓	↑	negative	→ (↑)	↑
Corticosteroid-induced osteopenia					
Cancellous	↓	?	negative	→	↑↓ [a]
Acromegaly					
Cortical	↓	↓	o	?	(↑)
Cancellous	?	?	?	→	?

Adapted from Eriksen, *et al.* (18).
[a]Ac.f may change with the duration of disease.
[b]Dt.BRU may be negative when accompanied by postmenopausal status.
Arrows indicate the direction of change. Entries in parentheses indicate preliminary or controversial data for which confirmation is, at the present time, lacking. Question marks indicate that the direction of change is unknown.

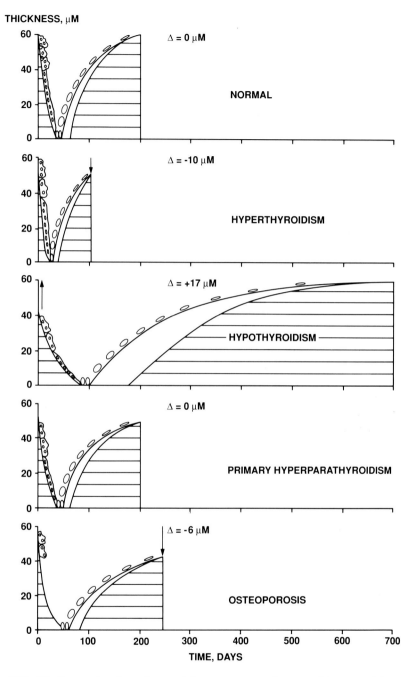

FIG. 19. Reconstruction of remodeling sequences in normal bone metabolism and in different metabolic bone diseases. Note the shorter duration and negative bone balance (Δ) in hyperthyroidism, the increased duration and positive bone balance in hypothyroidism, the preservation of bone balance in primary hyperparathyroidism, and the modest prolongation and negative bone balance in osteoporosis. Adapted from Eriksen *et al.* (16, 29, 50, 53, 59).

best explained by imbalances between resorption and formation at the endosteal surfaces of cortical bone.

In cancellous bone, Darby *et al.*(42) found reductions in the mean wall thickness in osteoporotic subjects but could not demonstrate any significant differences in other histomorphometric indices. Eriksen *et al.* (43) found a significant negative bone balance per remodeling cycle in osteoporotic subjects, whereas Steiniche *et al.*(44) were unable to identify any significant remodeling imbalance. However, no age-matched samples were used as reference in either of the latter two studies.

In a recent study by Eriksen *et al.* (16), data from bone biopsy samples obtained from 58 osteoporotic subjects were compared with those from 26 age- and sex-matched normal subjects. Osteoporotic subjects exhibited a slight, although nonsignificant, increase in erosion depth but a significant increase in the rate of resorption. Activation frequency was also increased but not significantly. The most marked difference between the two groups was a pronounced reduction in mean wall thickness in the osteoporotic group as compared with the control group (35 mm versus 50 mm, respectively), leading to a pronounced remodeling imbalance. When bone balance (as mean wall thickness minus erosion depth) in normal and osteoporotic subjects was compared, the latter in most cases exhibited negative balance, whereas all normal subjects exhibited balance values near zero.

Cohen-Solal *et al.*(45) also recently found a similar profound reduction in the mean wall thickness in osteoporotic subjects. In their study, however, resorption indices were similar to those in control subjects.

The histologic findings of these studies suggest that normal osteoblasts are able to "balance" resorptive activity. However, in osteoporotic subjects, every resorption cavity is not completely refilled, leading to pronounced thinning of trabeculae and eventual removal of the thin trabecular structures by perforative resorption (Figs. 10, 12b, and 12c).

OSTEOMALACIA

The histologic diagnosis of osteomalacia is based on the concurrent presence of two abnormalities: increased mineralization lag time (the time necessary for newly deposited matrix to mineralize) and increased osteoid width (41,46,47). Most osteomalacic states are also characterized by bone changes caused by compensatory secondary hyperparathyroidism.

Osteomalacia has been subdivided into three forms (Fig. 20) (48): a mild form dominated by secondary hyperparathyroidism and characterized by normal osteoid thickness and increased bone turnover; an intermediate form histologically characterized by areas with increased osteoid thickness mixed with areas with increased resorption; and an advanced form, also called "end-stage" osteomalacia, characterized by low turnover and the presence of flattened osteoblasts lining thick osteoid seams.

THYROID DISORDERS

Hyperthyroidism produces a state of increased bone turnover with a negative BRU balance, making this disease a state of accelerated and irreversible bone loss in cancellous bone (Fig. 19) (49,50). Trabecular thinning in combination with increased bone turnover leads to increased perforative resorption. Cortical porosity is increased, and increased endosteal resorption results in cortical thinning.

In contrast with hyperthyroidism, hypothyroidism is characterized by a profound reduction in bone turnover. At the BRU level, a significant positive balance is achieved in cancellous bone (Fig. 19), but, as a result of the low turnover, only small increases in bone mass occur (29). Although the mineralization lag time is increased, this does not reflect a mineralization defect but rather the profound prolongation of the formation period. In cortical bone, both erosion depth and wall thickness are increased, with a resulting positive bone balance at the BRU level(12).

PRIMARY AND SECONDARY HYPERPARATHYROIDISM

Bone turnover is increased in primary hyperparathroidism (51-53). Wall thickness is reduced in cancellous bone, as is erosion depth (53). Bone balance at the level of individual BRUs is therefore preserved (Fig. 19), at least in younger individuals (53). In older women, a slightly negative bone balance has been demonstrated(54).

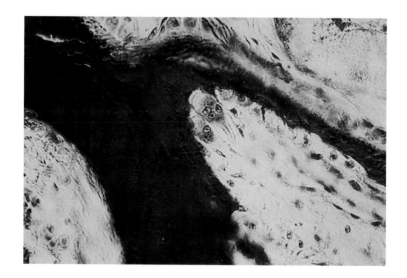

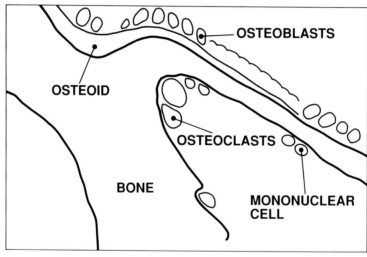

FIG. 20. The three stages of osteomalacia as seen in bone biopsy samples. The mild form is characterized by secondary hyperparathyroidism (i.e., accumulation of osteoid, high osteoclastic activity) (**a**); the intermediate form, characterized by secondary hyperparathyroid changes and marrow fibrosis (**b**); and the advanced form ("end-stage" osteomalacia), by flattened osteoblasts lining thick osteoid seams covering the bone surface (**c**). a, Masson-Trichrome, x 500; b,c, Masson-Trichrome, x 200.

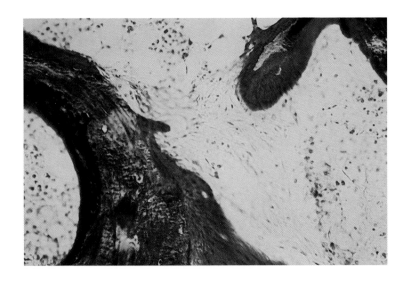

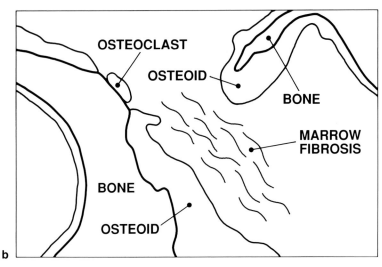

FIG. 20. Continued.

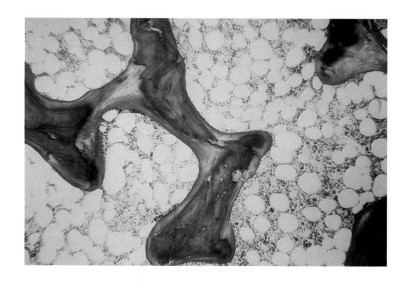

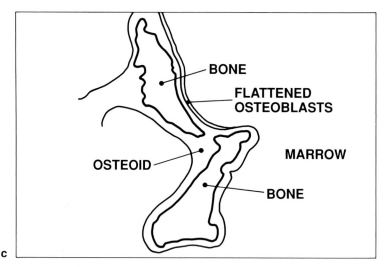

c

FIG. 20. Continued.

In cortical bone, wall thickness and erosion depth are similar to those in age-matched normal subjects (12), but the increase in bone turnover leads to increased cortical porosity and thinning of the trabecular elements (Fig. 21).

Secondary hyperparathyroidism is characterized primarily by increased turnover in which trabeculae may be penetrated by tunneling resorption, associated with marrow fibrosis. Some diseases accompanied by secondary hyperparathyroidism, such as postgastrectomy syndrome, may also display low measured bone density. This combination of secondary hyperparathyroidism and suppressed bone formation leads to severe osteopenia.

CORTICOSTEROID-INDUCED OSTEOPENIA

The acute effects of corticosteroid administration on bone remodeling are dominated by alterations similar to those seen in secondary hyperparathyroidism (55). In long-standing corticosteroid-induced osteopenia, a clear reduction of wall thickness in cancellous bone has been demonstrated (56), as is consistent with the suppression of bone formation (57), and bone turnover is decreased (58).

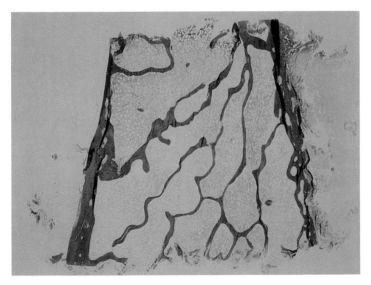

FIG. 21. Bone biopsy section from a patient with primary hyperparathyroidism. Cortical thinning is evident. Trabeculae are also thinned but with few perforations, thus, connectivity is maintained. Masson-Trichrome, x 25.

References

1. Frost HM. Tetracycline-based histological analysis of bone re-modeling. *Calcif Tissue Res* 1969;3:211-237.
2. Parfitt AM. The physiologic and clinical significance of bone his-tomorphometric data. In: Recker RR, ed. *Bone histomorphometry: techniques and interpretation.* Boca Raton, FL: CRC Press; 1983:143-223.
3. Eriksen EF. Normal and pathological remodeling of human tra-becular bone: three-dimensional reconstruction of the remodel-ing sequence in normals and in metabolic bone disease. *Endocr Rev* 1986;7:379-408.
4. Jaworski ZF, Lok E. The rate of osteoclastic bone erosion in haversian remodeling sites of adult dog's rib. *Calcif Tissue Res* 1972;10:103-112.
5. Kragstrup J, Melsen F. Three-dimensional morphology of tra-becular bone osteons reconstructed from serial sections. *Metab Bone Dis Relat Res* 1983;5:127-130.
6. Parfitt AM. The physiologic and pathogenetic significance of bone histomorphometric data. In: Coe FL, Favus MJ, eds. *Disorders of bone and mineral metabolism.* New York: Raven Press; 1992:475-489.
7. Mosekilde Li. Consequences of the remodelling process for ver-tebral trabecular bone structure: a scanning electron microscopy study (uncoupling of unloaded structures). *Bone Miner* 1990;10:13-35.
8. Frost HM. Some effects of basic multicellular unit-based remodelling on photon absorptiometry of trabecular bone. *Bone Miner* 1989;7:47-65.

9. Jerome CP. Estimation of bone mineral density variation associated with changes in turnover rate. *Calcif Tissue Int* 1989;44:406-410.

10. Melsen F, Nielsen HE, Christensen P, Mosekilde Li, Mosekilde Le. Some relations between photon-absorptiometric and histomorphometric measurements of bone mass in the forearm. In: Mazess RB, ed. *Proceedings, Fourth International Conference on Bone Measurement*, Ontario, Canada, June 1-3,1978. Bethesda,MD: National Institutes of Health; 1980; Publication No. 80-1938;45-50.

11. Eriksen EF, Riggs BL, Kumar R. Osteoporosis: recent concepts and approaches to treatment. *New Dev Med* 1987;2:11-23.

12. Broulik P, Kragstrup J, Mosekilde L, Melsen F. Osteon cross-sectional size in the iliac crest. *APMIS* 1982;90:339-344.

13. Eriksen EF, Mosekilde L, Melsen F. Trabecular bone resorption depth decreases with age: differences between normal males and females. *Bone* 1985;6:141-146.

14. Dempster DW, Shane E, Horbert W, Lindsay R. A simple method for correlative light and scanning electron microscopy of human iliac crest bone biopsies: qualitative observations in normal and osteoporotic subjects. *J Bone Miner Res* 1986;1:15-21.

15. Mosekilde Li, Søgaard C. Consequences of the remodeling process for vertebral structure and strength. In: Christiansen C, Overgaard K, eds. *Osteoporosis 1990. Proceedings of the Third International Symposium on Osteoporosis*, Copenhagen, Denmark, October 14-20, 1990. Copenhagen: Osteopress ApS; 1990:607-609.

16. Eriksen EF, Hodgson SF, Eastell R, Cedel SL, O'Fallon WM, Riggs BL. Cancellous bone remodeling in type I (postmenopausal) osteoporosis: quantitative assessment of rates of formation, resorption, and bone loss at tissue and cellular levels. *J Bone Miner Res* 1990;5:311-319.

17. Riggs BL, Wahner HW, Dunn WL, Mazess RB, Offord KP, Melton LJ III. Differential changes in bone mineral density of the appendicular and axial skeleton with aging. Relationship to spinal osteoporosis. *J Clin Invest* 1981;67:328-335.

18. Eriksen EF, Vesterby A, Kassem M, Melsen F, Mosekilde Le.

Bone remodeling and bone structure. In: Mundy GR, Martin TJ, eds. *Physiology and pharacology of bone.* New York: Springer Verlag; 1993: 67-109.

19. Riggs BL, Hodgson SF, O'Fallon WM, Chao EYS, Wahner HW, Muhs JM, *et al.* Effect of fluoride treatment on the fracture rate in postmenopausal women with osteoporosis. *N Engl J Med* 1990; 332:802-809.

20. Neer R, Slovik D, Daly M, Lo C, Potts J, Nussbaum S. Treatment of postmenopausal osteoporosis with daily parathyroid hormone plus calcitriol. In:Christiansen C, Overgaard K, eds. *Osteoporosis 1990. Proceedings of the Third International Symposium on Osteoporosis*, Copenhagen, Denmark, October 14-20, 1990. Copenhagen: Osteopress ApS; 1990:1314-1317.

21. Lindsay R, Hart DM, Forrest C, Baird C. Prevention of spinal osteoporosis in oophorectomized women. *Lancet* 1980;2:1151-1154.

22. Storm T, Thamsborg G, Steiniche T, Genant HK, Sørensen OH. Effect of intermittent cyclical etidronate therapy on bone mass and fracture rate in women with postmenopausal osteoporosis. *N Engl J Med* 1990; 322:1265-1271.

23. Munk-Jensen N, Pors Nielsen S, Obel EB, Bonne Eriksen P. Reversal of postmenopausal vertebral bone loss by oestrogen and progestogen: a double blind placebo controlled study. *BMJ* 1988;296:1150-1152.

24. Marie PJ, Rasmussen H, Kuntz D, Gueris J, Caulin F. Treatment of postmenopausal osteoporosis with phosphate and intermittent calcitonin. In: Christiansen C, Arnaud CD, Nordin BEC, Parfitt AM, Peck WA, Riggs BL, eds. *Osteoporosis: Proceedings of the Copenhagen International Symposium on Osteoporosis*, Copenhagen, Denmark, June 3-8, 1984. Glostrup, Denmark: Department of Clinical Chemistry of Glostrup Hospital; 1984:575 -579.

25. Eriksen EF, Melsen F, Mosekilde L Reconstruction of the resorptive site in iliac trabecular bone: a kinetic model for bone resorption in 20 normal individuals. *Metab Bone Dis Relat Res* 1984;5:235-242.

26. Parfitt AM, Drezner MK, Glorieux FH, Kanis JA, Malluche H,

Meunier PJ, *et al.* Bone histomorphometry: standardization of nomenclature, symbols, and units. Report of the ASBMR histomorphometry nomenclature committee. *J Bone Miner Res* 1987;2:595-610.

27. Vesterby A. Star volume of marrow space and trabeculae in iliac crest: sampling procedure and correlation to star volume of first lumbar vertebra. *Bone* 1990;11:149-155.

28. Gundersen HJG, Bagger P, Bendtsen TF, Evans SM, Korbo L, Marcussen N, *et al.* The new stereological tools: dissector, fractionator, nucleator and point sampled intercepts and their use in pathological research and diagnosis. *APMIS* 1988;96:857-881.

29. Eriksen EF, Mosekilde L, Melsen F. Kinetics of trabecular bone resorption and formation in hypothyroidism: evidence for a positive balance per remodeling cycle. *Bone* 1986;7:101-108.

30. Charles P, Eriksen EF, Mosekilde L, Melsen F, Jensen FT. Bone turnover and balance evaluated by a combined calcium balance and [47]calcium kinetic study and dynamic histomorphometry. *Metabolism* 1987;36:1118-1124.

31. Arlot M, Edouard C, Meunier PJ, Neer RM, Reeve J. Impaired osteoblast function in osteoporosis: comparison between calcium balance and dynamic histomorphometry. *BMJ* 1984;289:517-520.

32. Pirok DJ, Ramser JR, Takahashi H, Villanueva AR, Frost HM. Normal histological, tetracycline and dynamic parameters in human, mineralized bone sections. *Henry Ford Hosp Med Bull* 1966;14:195-218.

33. Garrahan NJ, Mellish RWE, Compston JE. A new method for the two-dimensional analysis of bone structure in human iliac crest biopsies. *J Microsc* 1986;142:341-349.

34. Frost HM. The regional acceleratory phenomenon: a review. *Henry Ford Hosp Med J* 1983;31:3-9.

35. Frost HM. The biology of fracture healing. An overview for clinicians. Part I. *Clin Orthop* 1989;248:283-293.

36. Bartley MH Jr, Arnold JS, Haslam RK, Jee WSS. The relationship of bone strength and bone quantity in health, disease, and aging. *J Gerontol* 1966;21:517-521.

37. Parfitt AM. Trabecular bone architecture in the pathogenesis and prevention of fracture. *Am J Med* 1987;82 (suppl.1B): 68-72.

38. Mosekilde Li, Mosekilde Le. Sex differences in age-related changes in vertebral body size, density and biomechanical competence in normal individuals. *Bone* 1990;11:67-73.

39. Mosekilde Li, Mosekilde Le. Normal vertebral body size and compressive strength: relations to age and to vertebral and iliac trabecular body compressive strength. *Bone* 1986;7:207-212.

40. Delmas PD, Demiaux B, Arlot MA, Edouard C, Malaval L, Meunier PJ. Relationship between bone histomorphometric parameters and biochemical markers of bone turnover. In: Takahashi HE, ed. *Bone morphometry, Proceedings of the Fifth International Congress on Bone Morphometry.* Niigata, Japan, July 24-29, 1988. Niigata, Japan: Nishimura; 1990:488.

41. Parfitt AM, Rao DS, Stanciu J, Villanueva AR, Kleerekoper M, Frame B. Irreversible bone loss in osteomalacia. Comparison of radial photon absortiometry with iliac bone histomorphometry during treatment. *J Clin Invest* 1985;76:2403-2412.

42. Darby AJ, Meunier PJ. Mean wall thickness and formation periods of trabecular bone packets in idiopathic osteoporosis. *Calcif Tissue Int* 1981; 33:199-204.

43. Eriksen EF, Mosekilde L, Melsen F. Effect of sodium fluoride, calcium phosphate, and vitamin D_2 on trabecular bone balance and remodeling in osteoporotics. *Bone* 1985;6:381-389.

44. Steiniche T, Hasling C, Charles P, Eriksen EF, Melsen F, Mosekilde L. A randomized study on the effects of estrogen/gestagen or high dose calcium on trabecular bone remodeling in postmenopausal osteoporosis. *Bone* 1989;10:313-320.

45. Cohen-Solal ME, Shih MS, Lundy MW, Parfitt AM. A new method for measuring cancellous bone erosion depth: application to the cellular mechanisms of bone loss in postmenopausal osteoporosis. *J Bone Miner Res* 1991; 6:1331-1338.

46. Melsen F, Mosekilde Le. Trabecular bone mineralization lag time determined by tetracycline double-labeling in normal and certain pathological conditions. *APMIS* 1980;88:83-88.

47. Eriksen EF, Steiniche T, Mosekilde Le, Melsen F. Histomorphometric analysis of bone in metabolic bone disease. *Endocrinol Metab Clin North Am* 1989; 18:919-954.

48. Parfitt AM. Osteomalacia and related disorders. In: Avioli LV, Krane SM, eds. *Metabolic bone disease and clinically related disorders.* 2nd ed. Philadelphia: WB Saunders; 1990:329-396.

49. Melsen F, Mosekilde L. Morphometric and dynamic studies of bone changes in hyperthyroidism. *APMIS* 1977;85:141-150.

50. Eriksen EF, Mosekilde L, Melsen F. Trabecular bone remodeling and bone balance in hyperthyroidism. *Bone* 1985;6:421-428.

51. Meunier P, Vignon G, Bernard J, Edouard C, Courpron P, Porte J. La lecture quantitative de la biopsie osseuse, moyen de diagnostic et d'étude de 106 hyperparathyroidies primitives, secondaires et paranéoplasiques (Quantitative reading of the bone biopsy as a means for the diagnosis and study of 106 cases of primary, secondary and paraneoplastic hyperparathyroidism). *Rev Rhum Mal Osteoartic* 1972; 39:635-644.

52. Melsen F, Mosekilde L, Christensen MS. Interrelationships between bone histomorphometry, S-iPTH and calcium-phosphorus metabolism in primary hyperparathyroidism. *Calcif Tissue Res* 1977;24 (suppl.):R16(abst).

53. Eriksen EF, Mosekilde L, Melsen F. Trabecular bone remodeling and balance in primary hyperparathyroidism. *Bone* 1986;7:213-221.

54. Christiansen P, Steiniche T, Mosekilde Le, Hessov I, Melsen F. Primary hyperparathyroidism: changes in trabecular bone remodeling following surgical treatment–evaluated by histomorphometric methods. *Bone* 1990; 11:75-79.

55. Findling JW, Adams ND, Lemann J Jr, Gray RW, Thomas CJ, Tyrrell JB. Vitamin D metabolites and parathyroid hormone in Cushing's syndrome: relationship to calcium and phosphorus homeostasis. *J Clin Endocrinol Metab* 1982;54:1039-1044.

56. Dempster DW, Arlot MA, Meunier PJ. Mean wall thickness and formation periods of trabecular bone packets in corticosteroid-induced osteoporosis. *Calcif Tissue Int* 1983;35:410-417.

57. Melsen F, Nielsen HE. Osteonecrosis following renal allotrans-
    plantation. *APMIS* 1977;85:99-104.
58. Bressot C, Meunier PJ, Chapuy MC, Lejeune E, Edouard C,
    Darby AJ. Histomorphometric profile, pathophysiology and
    reversibility of corticosteroid-induced osteoporosis. *Metab
    Bone Dis Relat Res* 1979; 1:303-311.
59. Eriksen EF, Gundersen HJG, Melsen F, Mosekilde L.
    Reconstruction of the formative site in iliac trabecular bone in
    20 normal individuals. A kinetic model for matrix and mineral
    apposition. *Metab Bone Dis Relat Res* 1984; 5:243-252.

A

Activation, in bone remodeling, 13, 14
Activation frequency
 bone porosity and, 21-22
 calculation of, 40, 43
 changes, consequences of, 42, 47
 decreased, 21
 definition of, 15, 20
 in osteoporosis, 52, 54
 reversible bone loss and, 28
Age, bone mass and, 30-31
Antiresorptive therapies, 31

B

Basic muticellular unit (BMU), 2. *See also* Bone remodeling unit (BRU)
BFR/BV, 43-44
Birefringence, lamellar pattern and, 7-8
Bisphosphonates, bone density and, 21, 30, 31
BMU (basic muticellular unit), 2. *See also* Bone remodeling unit (BRU)
Bone, types of, 3. *See also* Cancellous bone; Cortical bone

Bone balance. *See also* Turnover
 calculation of, 46
 at each remodeling site, 46
 indices of, 44-47
 negative, 46, 51-54, 55
 in osteoporosis, 25-28, 51-54
 positive, 46, 52, 53, 55
 volume-referent, 44, 46
Bone biopsy
 indications for, 35
 procedures for, 35-37
 sample/section, criteria for, 37
Bone densitometry, 35
Bone formation. *See* Formation
Bone histology, definition of, 33
Bone histomorphometry. *See* Histomorphometry
Bone mass
 age-related loss of, 30-31
 changes in, 15, 21-28, 29-31
 irreversible changes in, 22-28
 mathematical modeling of, 29
 measurements of, 29-31
 remodeling changes and, 29
 reversible changes in, 21-22
 treatment-related changes in, 29-31
Bone mineral density, responses to treatment, 30
Bone modeling, 1
Bone porosity, 22, 55, 58
Bone remodeling. *See* Remodeling

Bone remodeling unit (BRU)
  bone balance changes and, 28, 52
  bone mass changes and, 29-31
  of cancellous bone, 6-7, 12
  of cortical bone, 3-4, 6, 12
  definition of, 2
  function and arrangement of, 13
  negative balance in, 22-23, 25, 28
  quantal activities of, 15, 20
  resorption-formation deficit in, 21
Bone resorption. *See* Resorption
Bone strength, bone structure and, 48-49
Bone structural unit (BSU)
  cortical osteon as, 3-4
  definition of, 2, 12
  trabecular osteon as, 7
Bone structure, bone strength and, 48-49
Bone surface/volume of trabecular bone (BS/BV), 40, 41, 44
BRs.R/BV, 40, 43-44, 46
BRU. *See* Bone remodeling unit (BRU)
BS/BV (bone surface/volume of trabecular bone), 40, 41, 44
BSU. See Bone structural unit (BSU)

C

Calcitonin, bone density and, 31
Calcium homeostasis
  in osteoporosis, 25
  remodeling and, 2
Cancellous bone
  activation frequency of, 43
  activation frequency of, in
    metabolic bone disease, 52
  bone remodeling unit of, 6-7
  decreased mass of, 21
  density of, 29
  erosion depth in, 46
  in forearm, 21, 23
  irreversible bone loss in, 22-28, 28
  lamellar pattern of, 7-9, 12
  metabolic activity of, 12
  in osteoporosis, 52, 54
  porosity of, activation frequency and, 21-22
  quantitative features of, 3, 5
  remodeling of, in metabolic bone disease, 52, 53
  remodeling sequence in, 14-15
  reversible bone loss in, 28
  structure of, 6-7, 9, 25-26
  trabeculae of, 4, 6
  wall thickness in, 46-47
Cartilage, longitudinal growth and, 1
Cell number, 39-41
"Closing cone" formation of new bone, 3-4, 12
Cortical bone
  activation frequency of, 43
  bone mass measurement of, 21, 23
  bone remodeling unit of, 3-4, 6
  density of, 29
  endosteal surface of, 5
  erosion depth in, 37, 45-46
  in forearm, 21, 23
  increased remodeling in, 21
  irreversible bone loss in, 22, 23, 28
  lamellar pattern of, 7-9, 12
  metabolic activity of, 12
  negative balance of, 46
  in osteoporosis, 51-52, 54

periosteal surface of, 5
porosity of.
    See Cortical porosity
positive balance of, 46
quantitative features of, 3, 5
remodeling of, in metabolic
    bone disease, 51-52, 54, 55,
    58
remodeling sequence in, 13-14
reversible bone loss in, 21
wall thickness in, 37, 45-46
Cortical osteon, 3-4, 12, 45-46
Cortical porosity
  changes in, 21, 22
  increased, 22, 23, 28
  in thyroid disorders, 55
Corticosteroid-induced osteopenia,
    59
Coupling, 20

D

Digitizing tablet, 35
1,25-Dihydroxyvitamin D_3,
    30, 31
Dissector techniques, 40

E

Endocortical thinning.
    See Endosteal surface, bone
    loss in
Endosteal surface
  bone loss in, 5-6, 22-23, 54
  of cortical bone, 5-6
  excessive resorption by, 22, 23
  resorption in, 28, 54, 55
EP. *See* Erosion period (EP)
Erosion depth
  bone balance and, 46

in cancellous bone, 46
changes, consequences of, 47
in cortical bone, 45-46
definition of, 37, 39, 45-46
Erosion period (EP)
  calculation of, 40
  in cancellous bone, 14
  in cortical bone, 13
  definition of, 13
Erosion rate (ER), 40, 43-44
Estrogen therapy, 21, 30, 31

F

Fluoride therapy
  bone density pattern and, 30
  bone formation stimulation and,
    31
  woven bone and, 10, 12, 14
Formation
  in bone remodeling, 13, 14
  indices of, 46
  rate of, 46
  in remodeling, 1-2
  stimulation therapies for, 31
Formation period (FP)
  calculation of, 40, 43
  in cortical bone, 13
  definition of, 13
Fracture risk, bone structure and,
    49-50
Functional periods, 43, 48. *See
    also* Erosion period;
    Formation period

G

Growth, of skeleton, 1
Growth plates, 1

H

Haversian system
  in cortical bone, 3-4
  increased canal diameter of, 22
Histomorphometry
  basis for evaluation, 33
  definition of, 33
  flow chart for, 36
  microscopic equipment for, 36, 38
  primary indices of, 39. *See also specific indices*
  procedure for, 35-37
  sample preparation techniques for, 35-37
  secondary indices of. *See also specific indices*
Hyperparathyroidism, 52, 53, 55-59
Hyperthyroidism, 21, 52, 53, 55
Hypothyroidism, 52, 53, 55

I

Ilium, anterior, 35, 38
Imbalance, 20
Immobilization, negative bone balance and, 20
Initial mineralization lag time, 14
Interlabel width, 39
Irreversible bone loss
  in cancellous bone, 22-25, 28
  in cortical bone, 22-23, 28

L

Labeled surface/erosion surface (LS/BS), 40, 41
Lamellae, 3-4, 46
Lamellar pattern, of cortical and cancellous bone, 7-9, 12
LS/BS (labeled surface/erosion surface), 40, 41

M

MAR (mineral appositional rate), 40, 43-44
Marrow star volume, 49-50
Mathematical modeling, of bone mass measurements, 29
Mechanical stimulation, of bone cells, 20
Menopause, 6
Metabolic bone diseases. *See also specific diseases*
  bone remodeling in, 51-59
Microtome, heavy-duty, 36, 38
Mineral appositional rate (MAR), 40, 43-44
Mineralization. *See* Formation
Mineralization lag time
  initial, 14
  in osteomalacia, 52, 54-55
  in thyroid disorders, 52, 55

O

OS/BS (osteoid-covered surface), 41
Osteoblasts
  activity of, 13-14, 46
  identification of, 41
  in osteomalacia, 55, 58
  recruitment of, 20
  in remodeling, 13, 14, 20
Osteoclasts, 13-14, 20, 41
Osteoid-covered surface (OS/BS), 41

Osteoid thickness (width)
  measurement of, 39, 40, 45
  in osteomalacia, 55
Osteomalacia
  bone remodeling in, 52, 53, 54-55
  stages of, 55, 56-58
Osteon
  cortical, 3-4, 6, 12, 37, 51
  trabecular, 6-7, 12, 15, 19
Osteopenia, corticosteroid-induced, 52, 59
Osteoporosis
  bone remodeling in, 51-54
  cancellous bone in, 25-28
  negative bone balance in, 25, 52, 53, 54

P

Paget's disease of bone, 10, 12, 14
Parathyroid hormone, 30, 31
Periosteal surface, of cortical bone, 5
Photon absorptiometry, for bone mass assessment, 29
Preosteoblasts, 13, 14, 15, 17, 37
Primary histomorphometric indices, 39, 47. *See also specific indices*
Primary hyperparathyroidism, 21, 52, 53, 55, 59
Progestin therapy, 30, 31
Prostaglandin E_2, 5

Q

Quantum concept, of bone remodeling, 15, 20

Quiescent period (QP), 43

R

Regional acceleratory phenomenon (RAP), 47-48
Remodeling
  activation-resorption-formation sequence of. *See Remodeling sequence*
  changes in, 29
  in corticosteroid-induced osteopenia, 52, 59
  definition of, 1-2, 12
  disturbances in, 2
  key indices of, 44-47
  in metabolic bone disease, 51-59
  in osteomalacia, 54-55, 56-58
  in osteoporosis, 51-54
  per unit of time. *See* Activation frequency
  quantum concept of, 15, 20
  traces of, 33
Remodeling cycle, 13
Remodeling period, 13, 20
  changes in duration of, 42
Remodeling sequence
  in cancellous bone, 7, 14-15, 16-19
  components of, 13, 14
  in cortical bone, 6, 13-14
  irreversible changes in bone mass and, 22-25
  reconstruction of, 44, 45, 48
  reversible changes in bone mass and, 21-22
Remodeling space, reduction of, 21
Resorption
  in bone remodeling, 13, 14

Resorption (*contd.*)
definition of, 1
on endosteal surfaces, 5-6, 23
indices of, 46
osteoclastic, 13
perforative, 23-24
Reversible bone loss, 21, 28

S

Secondary derived histomorpho-
metric indices, 39-40, 48. *See
also specific indices*
Secondary hyperparathyroidism,
56-57, 59
Skeletal growth, definition of, 1
Stains, for bone biopsy samples,
36, 41. *See also* Villaneueva
staining method
Steady state, 40
Structure widths, 39
Surface estimates, 39, 40-42

T

Tetracycline double labels, 33,
34, 36, 38, 39, 40, 43, 46
Thyroid disorders, bone remodeling in, 52, 53, 55
Thyroid hormone status, reduction of, 21
Thyrotoxicosis, 6

Tissue-level volume-referent
indices, 43-44
Total resorptive activity, 45
Trabeculae
in cancellous bone, 6
perforations of, 22-25, 27-28,
50
Trabecular bone.
See Cancellous bone
Trabecular osteon, 6-7, 12, 15, 19
Turnover. *See also* Bone balance
bone remodeling and, 29-31
tissue-level, index of, 46

V

Vertebral bodies, compressive
strength of, 49
Villaneueva staining method, 34,
36, 38
Volume-referent bone balance,
44, 46

W

Wall thickness
bone balance and, 44-45
in cancellous bone, 46-47
changes, consequences of, 47
in cortical bone, 37, 45-46
Wolff's Law, 1
Woven bone, 10-12, 14